The Ultimate Guide to Build Muscle & Stay Lean

The Bodybuilding Cookbook with Healthy and Delicious Recipes

BY: Valeria Ray

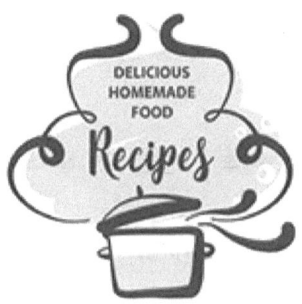

License Notes

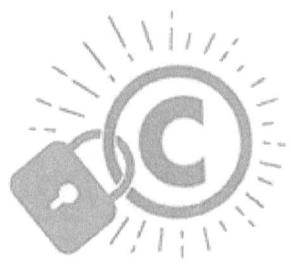

A Special Reward for Purchasing My Book!

Thank you, cherished reader, for purchasing my book and taking the time to read it. As a special reward for your decision, I would like to offer a gift of free and discounted books directly to your inbox. All you need to do is fill in the box below with your email address and name to start getting amazing offers in the comfort of your own home. You will never miss an offer because a reminder will be sent to you. Never miss a deal and get great deals without having to leave the house! Subscribe now and start saving!

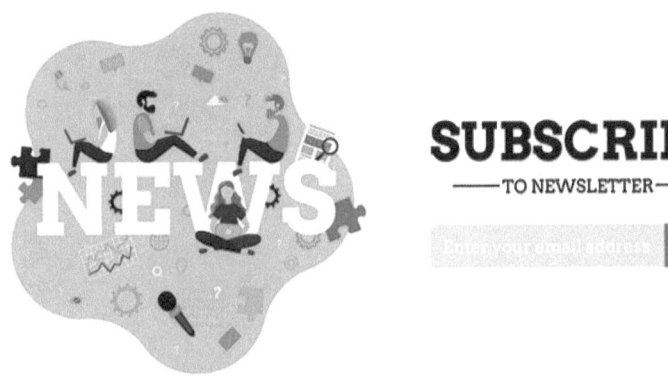

https://valeria-ray.gr8.com

Contents

Amazing Build Muscle Food

Recipes

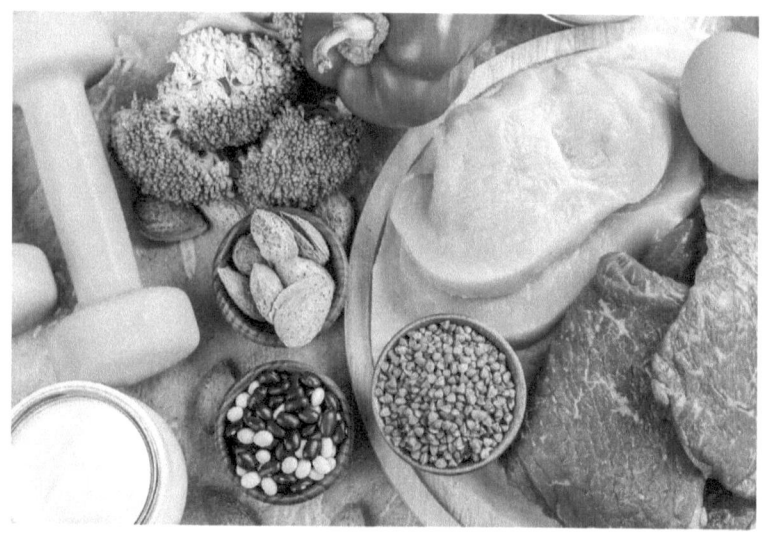

MMMMMMMMMMMMMMMMMMMMMMMMMMMMMMMMMM

Chapter I - Main Meals

MMMMMMMMMMMMMMMMMMMMMMMMMMMMMMMMMMMMM

(1) Zucchini Noodles with Turkey Bolognese

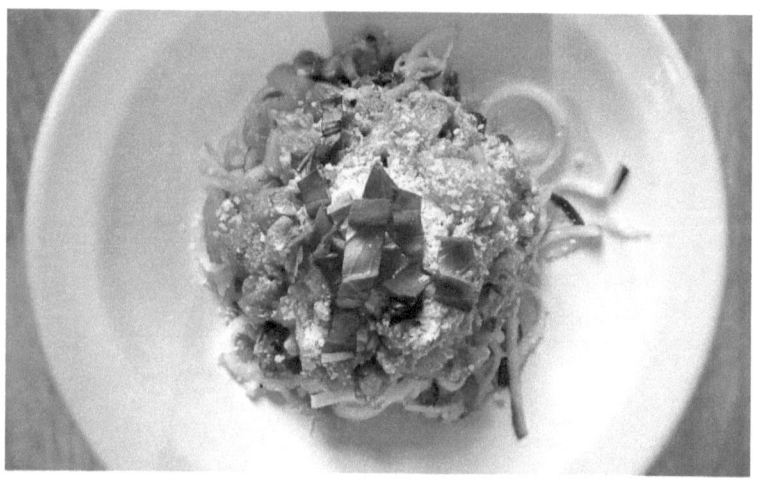

Zucchini is not only nutritious, but it is also a rich source of valuable fiber and is perfect for pairing with a protein-rich turkey Bolognese.

Yield: 4

Cooking Time: 35mins

List of Ingredients:

- 2 tablespoons virgin olive oil (divided)
- 1-pound extra-lean ground turkey
- ½ white onion (peeled, finely chopped)
- 1 celery stalk (finely diced)
- Salt and pepper
- ¼ teaspoons red pepper flakes
- 3 garlic cloves (minced)
- 1 (28 ounce) can crushed tomatoes
- 1 tablespoon store-bought tomato paste
- 1 (14 ½ ounce) can diced tomatoes
- 1 tablespoon dried oregano
- 1 teaspoon brown sugar
- 2 tablespoons fresh basil (chopped)
- 5 medium, fresh zucchinis
- 2 tablespoons Parmesan cheese (freshly grated)

MMMMMMMMMMMMMMMMMMMMMMMMMMMMMMMMMMMM

Methods:

1. Over moderately high heat, heat the olive oil in a skillet.

2. Add the ground turkey followed by the chopped onion and diced celery. Taste and season accordingly with a pinch of salt, a dash of pepper and red pepper flakes.

3. Cook the mixture for 8-10 minutes, until the turkey is sufficiently cooking. Use the back of a wooden spoon to break the turkey meat up as it cooks. Add the garlic and sauté for 60 seconds.

4. Add the crushed tomatoes to the skillet along with the tomato paste diced tomatoes, stir to combine and add the oregano and brown sugar.

5. Bring the mixture to boil before lowering the heat and reducing to a gently simmer for 15-20 minutes.

6. Scatter in the chopped basil and stir well to incorporate.

7. Next, using a spiralizer, prepare the zucchini noodles.

8. In a frying pan, over moderate to high heat, heat the oil. Add the spiralized zucchini and cook for 2-3 minutes, while occasionally stirring.

9. When the noodles are cooked, divide them between 4 serving bowls, top with the sauce and garnish with freshly grated Parmesan.

Nutrition per Serving

Cals 367 | Fat 11g | Carbs 37g | Protein 36g

(2) Grilled Steak and Veggies on a Bed of Arugula

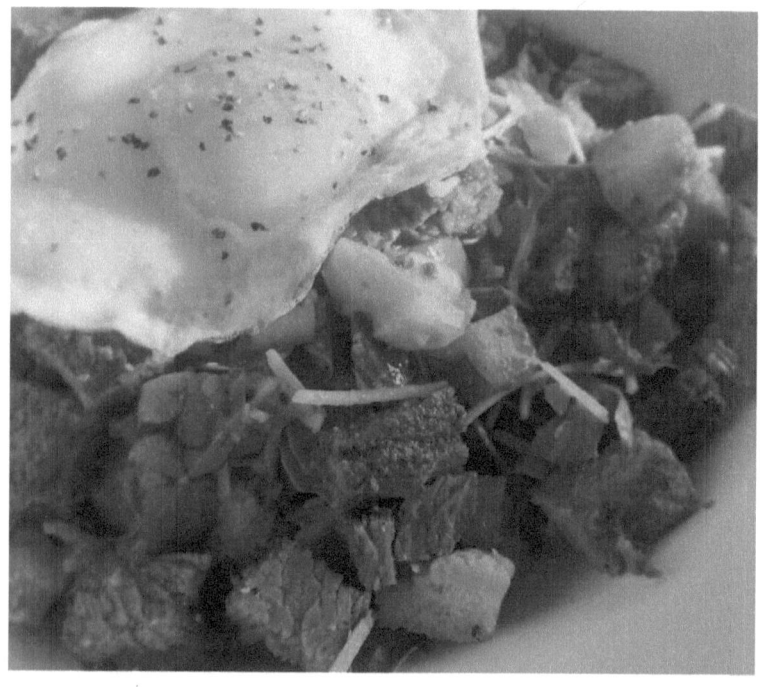

Low in carbs and high in protein with a host of vitamins. In fact, this is the perfect meal for any serious bodybuilder.

Yield: 1

Cooking Time: 40mins

List of Ingredients:

- 1 teaspoon onion powder
- 1 teaspoon garlic powder
- 1 teaspoon ground ginger
- 1 teaspoon chili powder
- 1 teaspoon paprika
- 1 teaspoon cayenne pepper
- 1 tablespoon light soy sauce
- 1 teaspoon brown sugar
- 4 ounces flank steak
- ½ cup red onion (peeled, sliced)
- ½ cup crimini mushrooms (sliced)
- 1 tablespoon olive oil
- Sea salt and black pepper
- 2 cups arugula (to serve)
- 1 tablespoon balsamic vinegar (to serve)

MMMMMMMMMMMMMMMMMMMMMMMMMMMMMMMMMM

Methods:

1. Add the onion and garlic powder, ginger, chili, paprika, cayenne, soy sauce, and brown sugar in a ziplock bag and shake to combine.

2. Add the steak to the marinade and gently massage to ensure that it is evenly coated. Allow to marinate for 20 minutes.

3. Lay the onions and mushrooms on a sheet of aluminum foil and drizzle with olive oil, and season sea salt and black pepper.

4. Remove the steak from the marinade, and very gently shake off any excess.

5. Transfer the steak to a grill and cook to your preferred level of doneness. After 5 minutes of grills, add the veggies on the foil to the grill and cook until caramelized.

6. Arrange the arugula on a plate, top with the grilled veggies, cooked steak, and drizzle with balsamic.

7. Enjoy.

Nutrition per Serving

Cals 417 | Fat 23g | Carbs 15g | Protein 34g

(3) Oysters with Spinach, Pine Nuts, and Feta

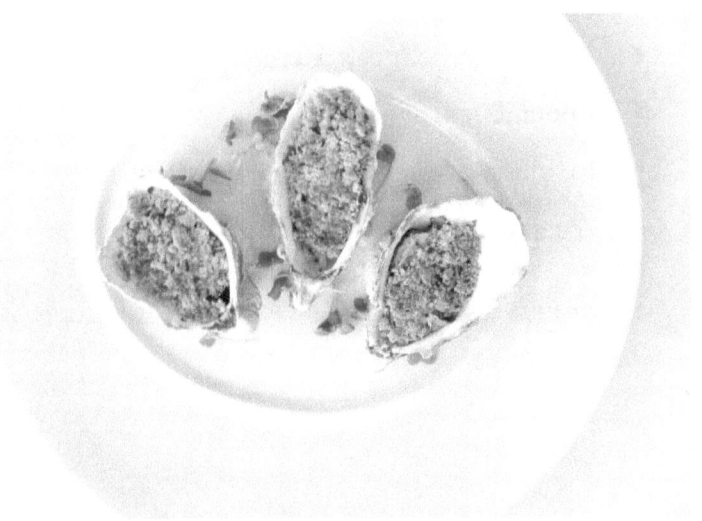

Oysters top the list of seafood that are rich in zinc, so eat them two or three times a week if you can, as they will help support your anabolic status. Zinc can help to support testosterone.

Yield: 2

Cooking Time: 1hour

List of Ingredients:

- 12 oysters
- 1 tablespoon virgin olive oil
- 1 small shallot (chopped)
- 2 cloves garlic (peeled, crushed)
- 2 pounds spinach leave
- 1 tablespoon pine nuts (toasted, chopped)
- ¼ cup feta cheese (crumbled)

MMMMMMMMMMMMMMMMMMMMMMMMMMMMMMMMM

Methods:

1. Preheat your broiler to moderate heat.

2. Shuck the oysters and set the bottom part of the shells to one side.

3. In a pan, heat the oil, add the shallot and garlic and sauté until translucent.

4. Add the spinach to the pan and sauté until it begins to wilt and is fork tender.

5. Throw the nuts in, stir and set to one side.

6. Arrange the oysters in the shells set aside earlier.

7. Spoon the spinach mixture over the top of the oysters.

8. Sprinkle with crumbled feta.

9. Transfer to the broiler and grill on the ½ shell for between 5-10 minutes. Cook them gently as this will avoid them being too chewy. As soon as their edges start to curl they should be taken off the heat.

Nutrition per Serving

Cals 308 | Fat 18g | Carbs 23g | Protein 23g

(4) Asian Salmon

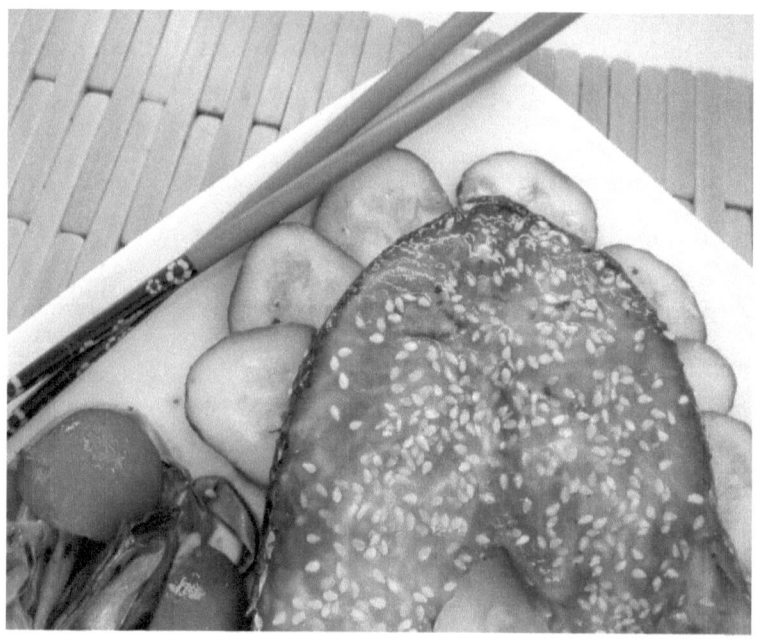

Salmon is one of the best fish for bodybuilders. It is high in Omega-3 which helps hardworking muscles beat inflammation. Plus, it tastes really good too!

Yield: 4

Cooking Time: 1hour

List of Ingredients:

Marinade:

- 3 tablespoons pure maple syrup
- ¼ cup soy sauce
- 3 tablespoons dark sesame oil
- ½ teaspoons Asian chili sauce
- 2 teaspoons Dijon mustard
- 2 scallions (chopped)
- 2 cloves garlic (peeled, minced)
- 2 tablespoons fresh ginger (finely chopped)
- 4 (4 ounce) wild salmon fillets (skin removed)

MMMMMMMMMMMMMMMMMMMMMMMMMMMMMMMMM

Methods:

1. In a bowl, make the marinade. Whisk the maple syrup with the soy sauce, sesame oil, chili sauce, and mustard. Stir in the scallions followed by the garlic and ginger.

2. Pour the marinade into an 8" square casserole dish.

3. Place the salmon fillets in the marinade, skin side facing upwards and allow to marinate for 30-60 minutes.

4. Preheat the main oven to 400 degrees F. Line a baking tray with aluminum foil.

5. Take the salmon out of the marinade and place on the prepared tray, skin facing downwards.

6. Bake in the preheated oven for 12-15 minutes, or until the fish flakes easily when using a fork and is sufficiently heated through.

Nutrition per Serving

Cals 274 | Fat 14.2g | Carbs 5g | Protein 29g

(5) Spanish Seafood Paella

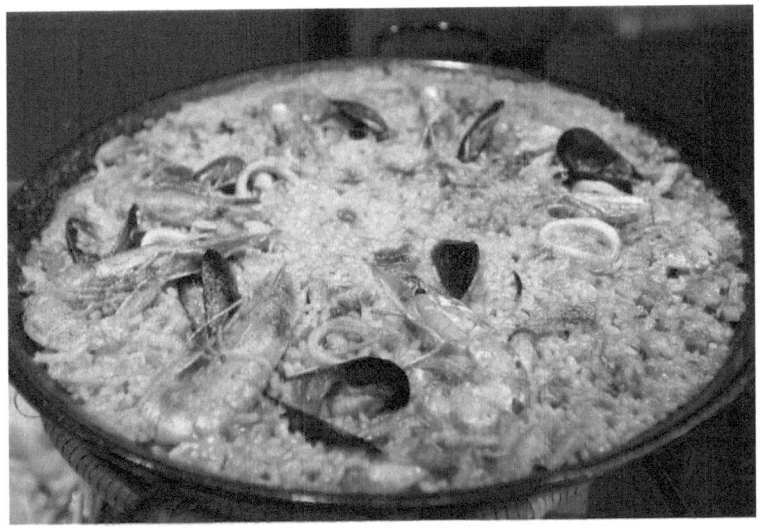

Give your body a well earned energy boost with the colorful and flavorsome paella.

Yield: 6

Cooking Time: 35mins

List of Ingredients:

- 2 tablespoons coconut oil
- ½ red onion (peeled, diced)
- 1 tablespoon garlic (peeled, minced)
- 1½ pounds chicken breast (chopped into bite-sized pieces)
- 1½ pounds small shrimp (peeled, deveined, chopped into bite-sized pieces)
- 1 tablespoon paprika
- Sea salt and black pepper
- 4 cups brown rice
- 2 large Roma tomatoes (diced)
- 2 cups chicken bone broth
- ½ teaspoons saffron
- Juice of 1 lemon
- ½ cup frozen peas
- Bunch of flat leaf parsley

MMMMMMMMMMMMMMMMMMMMMMMMMMMMMMMMMM

Methods:

1. Cook the rice according to the package instructions and set to one side.

2. Over moderately high heat, in a skillet, heat the coconut oil. Add the onion followed by the garlic. Using a wooden spoon stir until the onions are browned.

3. Add the chopped chicken and cook until the chicken is approximately ¾ cooked. At this stage, some of the chicken may be pink.

4. Add the shrimp and stir, cook, until the shrimp are ¾ cooked.

5. Add the paprika followed by a pinch of salt and a dash of pepper. Stir to combine.

6. Add the cooked brown rice, followed by the tomatoes. Reduce heat to moderate and stir to combine.

7. Pour in the broth and add the saffron. Simmer gently while stirring.

8. Cook for 3-4 minutes.

9. Stir in the lemon juice and the peas, stirring to combine.

10. Allow the paella to simmer for 5 minutes.

11. Garnish with parsley and serve.

Nutrition per Serving

Cals 401| Fat 8g | Carbs 41g | Protein 41g

(6) Barbecue Pork Chops

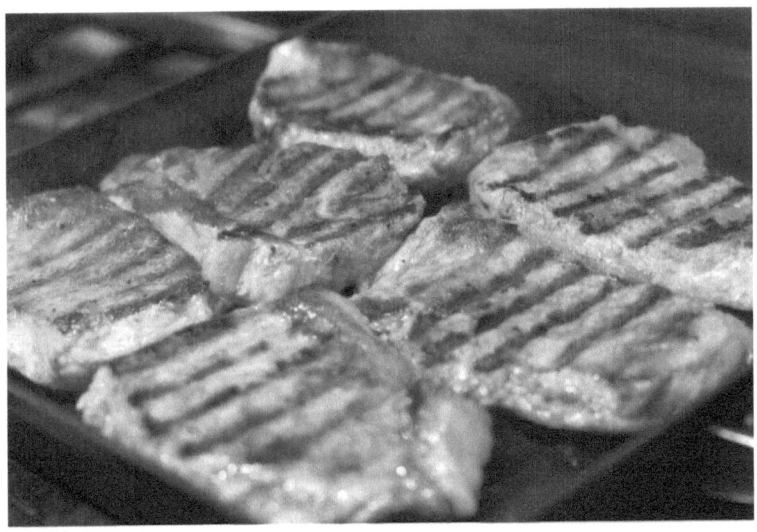

It's okay to eat pork once in a while. All you need to do is trim off any excess fat and choose the leanest cut.

Yield: 4

Cooking Time: 18mins

List of Ingredients:

- 1 tablespoon cider vinegar
- 1 tablespoon brown sugar
- 2 tablespoons Worcestershire sauce
- 4 tablespoons low-sugar ketchup
- 1 tablespoon chili powder
- 4 (9 ounce) pork chops* (trimmed of all fat)
- Nonstick cooking spray

MMMMMMMMMMMMMMMMMMMMMMMMMMMMMMMMMMMM

Methods:

1. In a bowl, make the marinade. Combine the cider vinegar, brown sugar, Worcestershire sauce, ketchup and chili powder and mix to combine. Transfer the marinade to a ziplock bag.

2. Using a sharp knife. Score the pork chops. The cuts need to be approximately ¼" deep.

3. Add the chops to the marinade.

4. Gently massage the bag to ensure the meat is evenly coated and transfer to the fridge for 4-6 to chill.

5. Spritz the grill with a high-temperature cooking spray and preheat.

6. Remove the porks chops from Zip lock bag and the marinade, shaking off any excess marinade and arrange on the grill.

7. Cook for approximately 5 minutes on each side until sufficiently cooked through.

*Weight of pork chops calculated on weighing before trimming

Nutrition per Serving

Cals 352 | Fat 18g | Carbs 5g | Protein 41g

(7) Mahi-Mahi Burger with Homemade Slaw

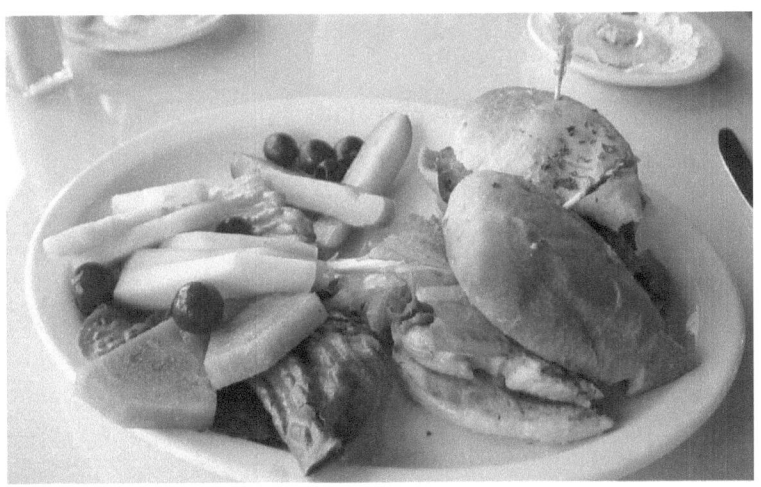

Incorporate fish into your weekly bodybuilding menu plan, and you will be reaping the rewards of its nutritional benefits.

Yield: 1

Cooking Time: 25mins

List of Ingredients:

- 3 ounces mahi-mahi

Dressing:

- 1 tablespoon cumin
- ½ cup fat-free Greek yogurt
- 1 tablespoon honey
- 2 tablespoons rice wine vinegar
- 1 teaspoon freshly squeezed lime juice
- 1 tablespoon jalapeno pepper (diced)
- 1 cup red cabbage (shredded)
- 1 teaspoon garlic (peeled, minced)
- ½ cup mango (peeled, pitted, sliced)
- ½ cup pineapple chunks (peeled)
- Pinch of salt
- Dash of pepper

To serve:

- 1 whole wheat thin bun
- 1 lettuce leaf
- ¼ avocado (peeled, pitted, sliced)

MMMMMMMMMMMMMMMMMMMMMMMMMMMMMMMMMMMMM

Methods:

1. On a grill, lightly grill the fish for a few minutes on each side. Set to one side.

2. Next, prepare the dressing. In a bowl, combine the cumin with the Greek yogurt, honey, vinegar, freshly squeezed lime juice, and jalapeno. Whisk to incorporate.

3. In a mixing bowl to make the slaw, combine the cabbage followed by the garlic, mango, and pineapple. Season with a pinch of salt and a dash of pepper.

4. Add approximately half of the dressing to the slaw. Set the remaining slaw to one side.

5. Spread a small amount of the set aside dressing onto the bottom half of the bun.

6. Next, layer the lettuce, followed by the slaw and cooked fish.

7. Finally, arrange the slices of avocado on top of the fish.

8. Top with the remaining half of the bun.

9. Enjoy.

Nutrition per Serving

Cals 557 | Fat 9g | Carbs 86g | Protein 34g

(8) Beef Jerk Casserole

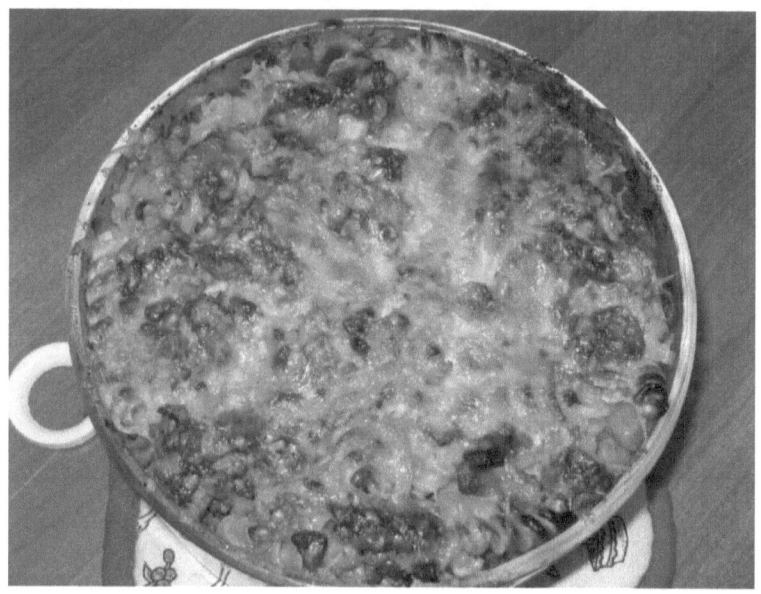

Obviously, there is a need to limit red meat in our diets, so when you do serve it, make it count, with this spicy jerk seasoned casserole dish.

Yield: 4

Cooking Time: 1hour 35mins

List of Ingredients:

- 1 tablespoon virgin olive oil
- 2 ½ pounds boneless, beef chuck (cut into 1" chunks)
- 1 yellow onion (peeled, diced)
- 4 carrots (cubed)
- 1 teaspoon garlic (minced)
- 2 cups salt-free chicken stock
- 2 teaspoons jerk sauce (any brand)
- 2 teaspoons Jamaican allspice seasoning
- ½ teaspoons cinnamon
- 1 tablespoon thyme
- 2 cups brown rice (cooked)

MMMMMMMMMMMMMMMMMMMMMMMMMMMMMMMMMM

Methods:

1. Preheat the main oven to 350 degrees F.

2. Over moderate to high heat, heat the oil in a Dutch oven. Add the chunks of beef and brown until cooked through all over, this will take around 8-10 minutes.

3. Add the onions followed by the carrots and garlic and stir to combine. Cook, while stirring for 3-4 minutes, until the onions are translucent.

4. Pour in the chicken broth and add the jerk sauce, seasoning, cinnamon and thyme. Stir and bring to boil.

5. Place a lid on the Dutch oven and transfer to the oven. Cook for between 60-90 minutes, until the beef, is cooked through and falls apart when shredded.

6. Remove the casserole from the oven. Serve immediately over brown rice.

Nutrition per Serving

Cals 480 | Fat 15g | Carbs 19g | Protein 57g

(9) Mac n Cheese

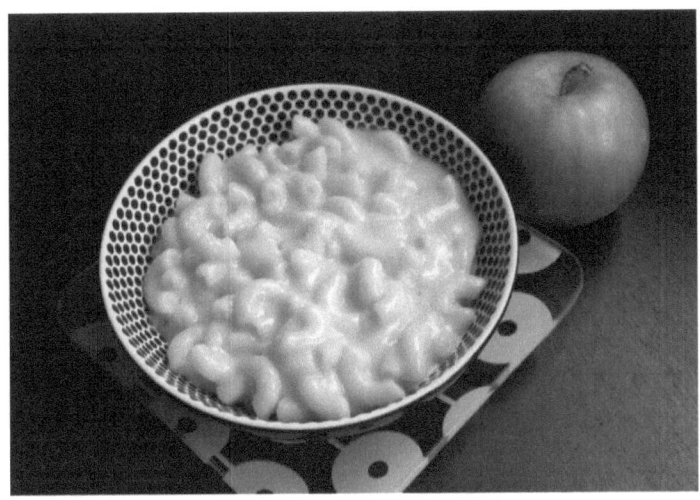

Plenty of protein and flavor with this Mac n Cheese and what's more your family will love it too!

Yield: 4

Cooking Time: 25mins

List of Ingredients:

- 8 ounces uncooked pasta
- 1 cup skimmed milk
- 2 teaspoons white pepper
- 1 ½ teaspoons onion powder
- 1 teaspoon garlic powder
- 2 cups fat-free cottage cheese
- ½ cup Greek yogurt
- 6 ounces low-fat white Cheddar
- ¼ cup Parmesan cheese (freshly grated)
- 2 tablespoons oat bran

MMMMMMMMMMMMMMMMMMMMMMMMMMMMMMMMMMMM

Methods:

1. Preheat the main oven to 420 degrees F.

2. Cook the pasta according to the package instructions, but deduct 2 minutes from the cooking time, remove from the heat and drain.

3. Return the drained pasta to the empty pot and add the milk followed by the white pepper, onion powder, garlic powder, cottage cheese, and yogurt.

4. Gradually stir in the white Cheddar and ½ of the grated Parmesan.

5. Transfer the mixture to a casserole dish.

6. Scatter the oat bran over the top along with the remaining Parmesan.

7. Bake in the preheated oven until the casserole bubbles and is golden.

Nutrition per Serving

Cals 472 | Fat 12g | Carbs 52g | Protein 40g

(10) Greek-Style Turkey Casserole

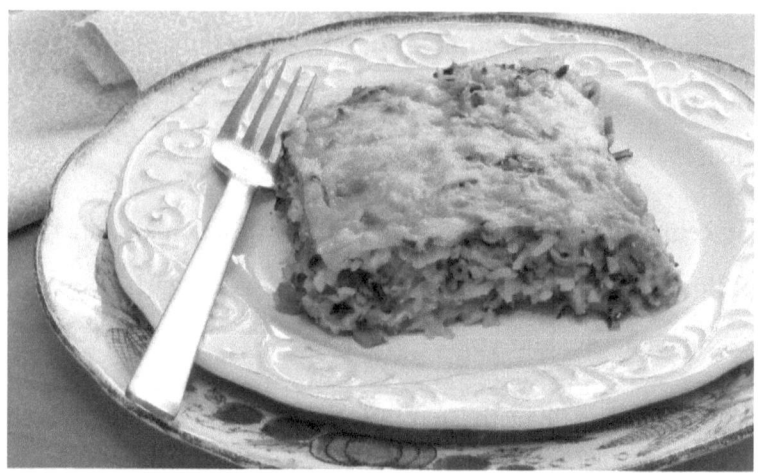

You can enjoy this casserole with friends and family safe in the knowledge that it is a super muscle-building meal, packed full of protein.

Yield: 6

Cooking Time: 1hour 20mins

List of Ingredients:

- 1 cup dry quinoa
- 2 cups chicken stock
- 1 tablespoon grapeseed oil
- ½ red onion (peeled, chopped)
- 1 tablespoon garlic (peeled, minced)
- 1¼ pounds 99% lean ground turkey
- ¼ teaspoons each of oregano, basil, and thyme
- ¾ cup Greek feta cheese
- 2 medium, free-range eggs
- 12 ounces frozen spinach (thawed, squeezed dry)
- ¼ cup fresh parsley (chopped)
- ¾ cup chicken stock (divided)
- ½ teaspoons sea salt
- ½ teaspoons white pepper
- Nonstick cooking spray6+-
- ¾ cup Italian four cheese blend

MMMMMMMMMMMMMMMMMMMMMMMMMMMMMMMMMMMM

Methods:

1. Preheat the main oven to 350 degrees F.

2. Cook the quinoa according the package instructions, switching the water for 2 cups of chicken broth. Allow to completely cool.

3. Add the grapeseed oil to a skillet over moderate heat and add the onion along with the garlic. Sauté for 3-4 minutes until translucent.

4. Add the turkey and sauté until no pink remains and the meat is sufficiently cooked through all over. Use the back of a wooden spoon to break the meat up.

5. In a mixing bowl, combine the turkey, cooked onion and garlic, oregano, basil, thyme, feta cheese, eggs, spinach, parsley and ¾ cup of chicken stock. Stir to incorporate and season.

6. Transfer the mixture to 13x9" casserole dish spritzed with nonstick spray and using the back of wooden spoon compact the mixture into an even layer.

7. Scatter with four cheese blend and bake in the preheated oven for 35-40 minutes, until the cheese bubbles and is golden.

8. Remove from the oven and transfer to the grill, grill for a few minutes until the surface of the bake is crunchy.

9. Allow to stand for 12-15 minutes.

10. Serve.

Nutrition per Serving

Cals 375 | Fat 15g | Carbs 15g | Protein 35g

(11) Lime Tilapia Curry

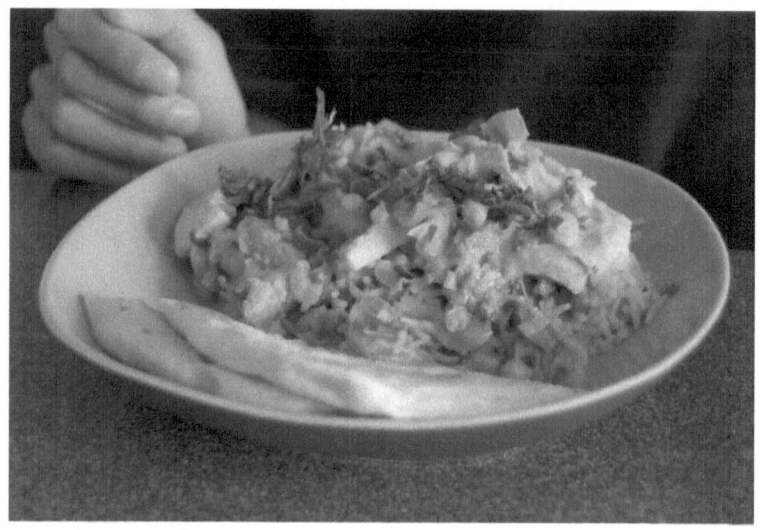

This fish is really low in fat but can be a little bland, so add a little tang and taste with lime juice and spices.

Yield: 4

Cooking Time: 25mins

List of Ingredients:

- 2 teaspoons ground oregano
- 2 teaspoons chili powder
- 2 teaspoons freshly ground black pepper
- 2 teaspoons garlic powder
- 4 tablespoons freshly squeezed lime juice
- 2teaspoons curry powder
- 4 tilapia fillets

MMMMMMMMMMMMMMMMMMMMMMMMMMMMMMMM

Methods:

1. In a bowl, combine the oregano, chili powder, black pepper, garlic powder, lime juice, and curry powder. Stir to combine the seasonings.

2. Season each of the fish fillets with an equal amount of the seasoning mix (1 teaspoon each).

3. Over moderate heat, in a skillet, cook for the fish for 2-3 minutes each side. Season with the remaining mix.

4. Cook for an additional 3-3 minutes, until the fish is sufficiently cooked through and flakes easily when using a fork.

Nutrition per Serving

Cals 141 | Fat 3g | Carbs 5g | Protein 24g

(12) Grilled Lamb Burger with Reduced Fat Dressing

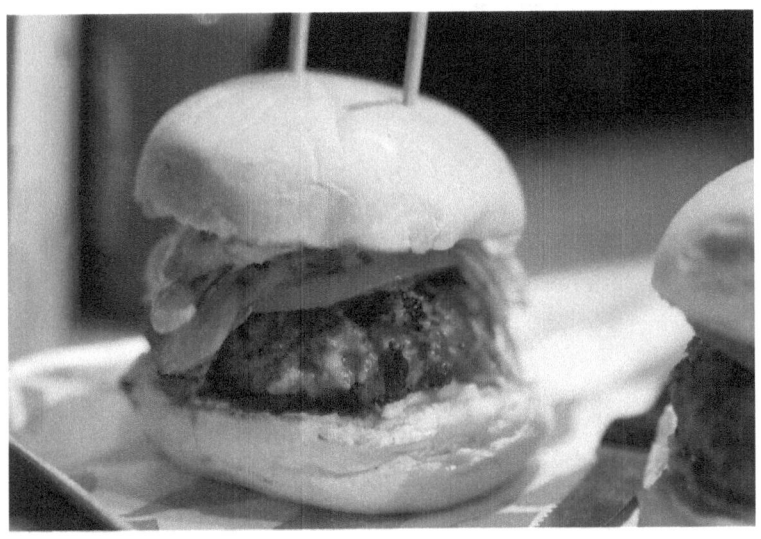

Red meat is an excellent source of protein and of course, super tasty. Make sure though, that you buy leaner cuts.

Yield: 2

Cooking Time: 35mins

List of Ingredients:

- 8 ounces lean, grass-fed lamb
- Pinch salt
- Dash black pepper

Dressing:

- ¼ cup reduced-fat sour cream
- 1 tablespoon sriracha
- 2 pinches dried parsley
- Juice of ¼ lemon
- To serve:
- 1 hamburger bun (split)
- 1 avocado (peeled, pitted, thinly sliced)
- ½ red onion (peeled, diced small)

MMMMMMMMMMMMMMMMMMMMMMMMMMMMMMMMMMMM

Methods:

1. Add the ground lamb to a bowl and season with salt and pepper. Mix to incorporate, using the back of a spoon to break the meat up.

2. Using clean hands divide the meat mixture evenly and shape 4 lamb patties.

3. In a grill, cook the patties until sufficiently cooked on both sides.

4. In the meantime, and while the patties cook, prepare the dressing.

5. In a bowl, combine the sour cream with the sriracha, parsley and freshly squeezed lemon juice and whisk until incorporated.

6. Lightly toast the hamburger burger bun.

7. Spoon the dressing on the bottom half of the toasted bun.

8. Arrange the slices of avocado on top of the dressing, in a fan shape.

9. Place the cooked patties on top of the avocado.

10. Scatter with red onions.

11. Top with the remaining half of the toasted bun.

12. Serve and enjoy.

Nutrition per Serving

Cals 480 | Fat 32g | Carbs 26g | Protein 23g

(13) Instant Pot Roast with Sweet Potatoes

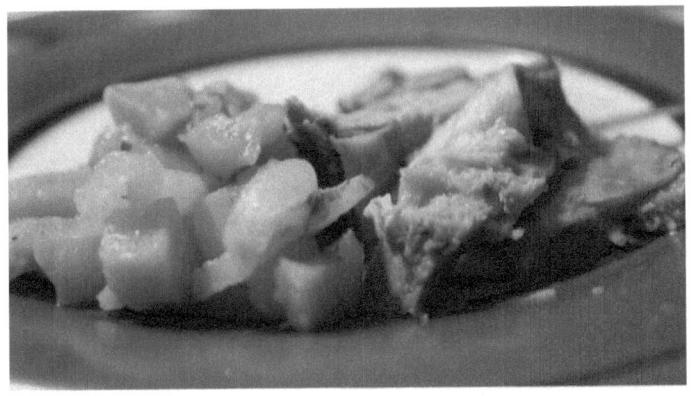

Cooking using an instant pot is a great way to keep the meat tender and moist. If you intend to hit the gym hard, then by including sweet potatoes in your diet you are providing your body with a good energy boost.

Yield: 4

Cooking Time: 1hour 15mins

List of Ingredients:

- 1 tablespoon virgin olive oil
- 2 pound lean roast eye round of beef
- 2 onions (peeled, sliced)
- 2 cups mushrooms (sliced)
- 2 garlic cloves (peeled, minced)
- 1 beef broth stock cube
- 1 tablespoon each of rosemary and thyme
- ½ tablespoons light soy sauce
- 1 tablespoon fish sauce
- Salt and pepper
- 4 sweet potatoes (cubed)
- 2 small carrots (sliced)
- 4 celery stalks (trimmed, finely diced)

MMMMMMMMMMMMMMMMMMMMMMMMMMMMMMMMM

Methods:

1. Set an instant pot to sauté and add the olive oil.

2. As soon as the oil is sufficiently hot, add the roast, flipping over every 60 seconds until the roast is evenly browned.

3. Remove the meat from the pot and put to one side.

4. To the instant pot, add the onions, followed by the mushrooms and garlic and sauté.

5. Add the broth cube and stir to combine.

6. Scatter in the rosemary and thyme and add the soy sauce along with the fish sauce. Season.

7. Add the roast beef and sweet potatoes to the pot cover the pot and cook for 45 minutes.

8. After this time, add the carrots followed by the celery. Replace the lid and cook for an additional 5 minutes.

9. After 5 minutes have elapsed, relieve the pressure.

10. As soon as the pressure has sufficiently reduced, remove the beef roast, and serve with the veggies.

Nutrition per Serving

Cals 5821 | Fat 13g | Carbs 41g | Protein 75g

(14) Hearty Slow-Cooked Bison Chili

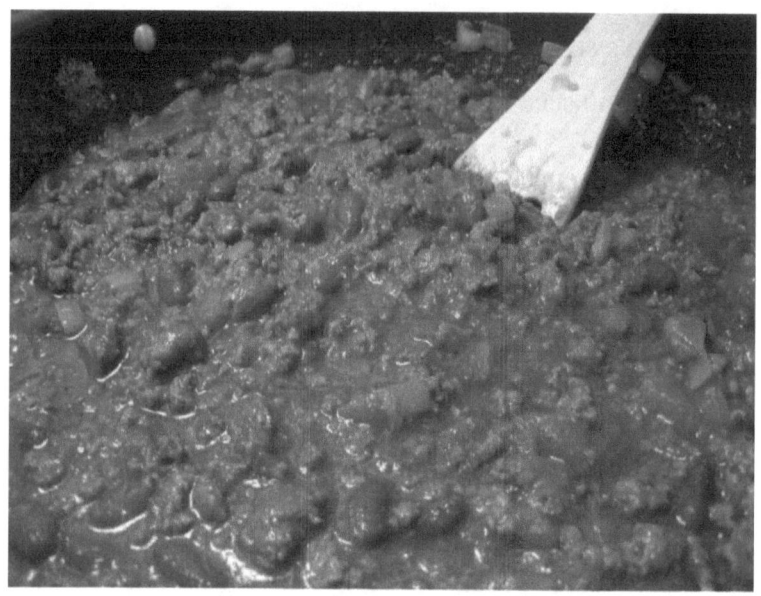

With approximately 35g of protein in every 6 ounce serving, bison really is a bodybuilder's dream food!

Yield: 10

Cooking Time: 6hours 10mins

List of Ingredients:

- 3 tablespoons virgin olive oil (divided)
- 4 cloves garlic (peeled, chopped, divided)
- 1½ pounds ground bison
- 1 red pepper (thinly sliced)
- 1 yellow pepper (cut into fine strips)
- 1 green pepper (cut into fine strips)
- 2 celery stalks (trimmed, finely diced)
- 2 onions (peeled, finely diced)
- Salt and black pepper
- 1 (14 ounce) can white beans
- 1 (14 ounce) can kidney beans
- 1 (28 ounce) can tomato sauce
- 1 cup water
- 1 tablespoon chili powder

MMMMMMMMMMMMMMMMMMMMMMMMMMMMMMMMMMMMM

Methods:

1. Over moderate heat, add 1 tablespoon of olive oil to a skillet and heat.

2. Add half of the garlic followed by the bison and cook, while continually stirring until the meat is no longer pink.

3. Transfer the mixture to a slow cooker and cook on low, for 3 hours.

4. When 3 hours has elapsed, heat the remaining oil in the skillet.

5. Add the remaining garlic and sauté until fragrant.

6. Add the veggies (red pepper, yellow pepper, green pepper, celery, and onions) along with a pinch of salt and a dash of pepper.

7. Transfer the veggie mixture to the slow cooker.

8. Add the white beans, kidney beans, tomato sauce, and water.

9. Add the chili powder and stir. Taste and season if needed.

10. On low heat, cook for 3 hours, until sufficiently cooked through.

11. Serve.

Nutrition per Serving

Cals 320 | Fat 15g | Carbs 24g | Protein 23g

Chapter II - Pre & Post - Workout Snacks

MMMMMMMMMMMMMMMMMMMMMMMMMMMMMMMMMMMM

(15) Turkey Pesto Roll-Ups

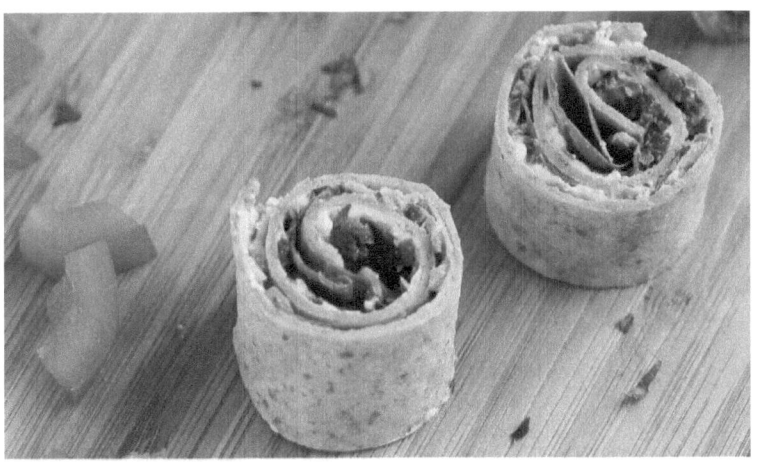

A heavy workout can often leave you feeling hungry; it can be easy to turn to fattening snacks and quickly undo all of your good work. Next time you have the post-workout munchies, reach for something low-carb, low-calorie but totally delicious like these turkey pesto roll-ups!

Yield: 18

Cooking Time: 10mins

List of Ingredients:

- 3 medium cucumbers (sliced into 18 long strips using a mandolin)
- ¼ cup organic green pesto
- 6 ounces smoked deli turkey breast (sliced into strips)
- 6 slices low-fat mozzarella (each sliced into 3 strips)
- ½ cup fresh baby spinach (sliced into thin strips)
- 1 red bell pepper (seeded, sliced into strips)

MMMMMMMMMMMMMMMMMMMMMMMMMMMMMMMMMMMMMM

Methods:

1. Pat the cucumber strips dry with kitchen paper.

2. Spread a teaspoon of pesto onto each slice of cucumber and divide the turkey breast, cheese, spinach, and pepper equally between the slices.

3. Roll up and secure with a toothpick if necessary. Enjoy!

Nutrition per Serving

Cals 50 | Fat 3g | Carbs 2.5g | Protein 4g

(16) Coconut and Tahini Energy Squares

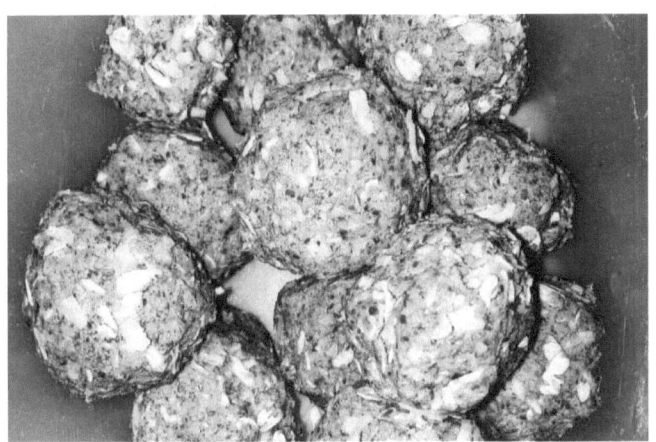

Tahini is a delicious sesame seed paste widely used in Mediterranean and Middle Eastern cooking; it brings rich nutty flavor as well as a good dose of protein and iron to these yummy coconut squares.

Yield: 20

Cooking Time: 1hour

List of Ingredients:

- Nonstick spray
- 1 cup shredded coconut
- 2 cups oats (old-fashioned variety)
- 1 cup mixed raw nuts
- ½ cup pitted dates (chopped)
- 1 cup mixed raw seeds
- 1½ cups organic tahini
- 1 cup raw honey
- 1 teaspoon pure vanilla essence

MMMMMMMMMMMMMMMMMMMMMMMMMMMMMMMMMM

Methods:

1. Preheat the main oven to 350 degrees F and spritz a (15x10") baking sheet with nonstick spray.

2. Add the coconut, oats, nuts, dates, and seeds to a bowl and toss to combine.

3. Add the tahini and honey to a small bowl. Stir to combine and then pop in the microwave for 60 seconds until runny. Stir in the vanilla essence.

4. Pour the tahini mixture over the oats and stir until the dry ingredients are well and evenly coated.

5. Press the mixture into the baking sheet and place in the oven for 15 minutes until browned and golden.

6. Set aside to cool completely before slicing into evenly sized squares.

Nutrition per Serving

Cals 295 | Fat 17.5g | Carbs 31g | Protein 6.5g

(17) Apricot and Raisin Chewy Bites

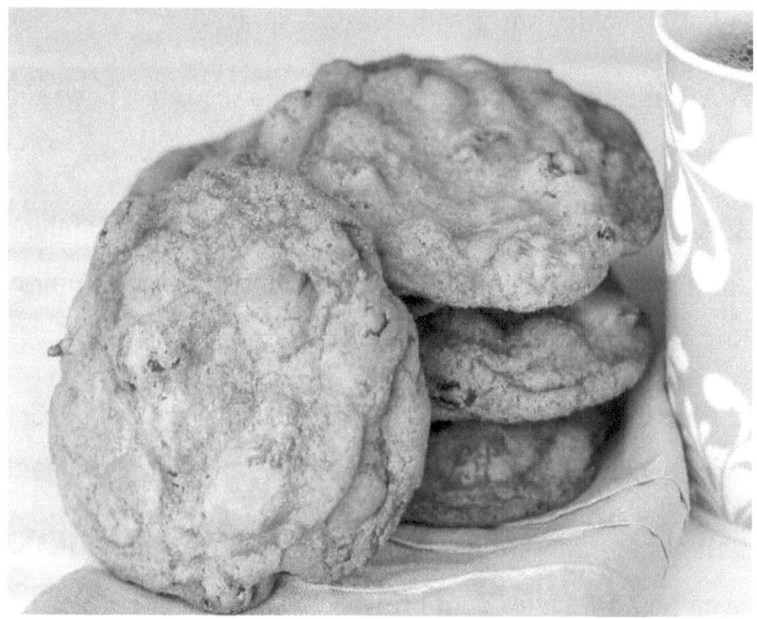

Each addictively chewy, sticky bite of these apricot and raisin treats is packed with protein and fibre making them the perfect pop-in-the-mouth fuel.

Yield: 25

Cooking Time: 45mins

List of Ingredients:

- ½ teaspoons cinnamon
- 1 cup raisins
- 1 cup almonds
- ½ cup shredded coconut
- 10 dried, chopped apricots

MMMMMMMMMMMMMMMMMMMMMMMMMMMMMMM

Methods:

1. Add the cinnamon, raisins, and almonds to a food processor, blitz for 3-4 minutes until your form a smooth paste.

2. Add the coconut and apricots, pulse until apricots are chopped into small pieces.

3. Cover your worktop with plastic wrap.

4. Turn the apricot dough out onto the plastic wrap. Place another piece of plastic wrap on top of the dough and press the mixture into a compact square.

5. Wrap tightly and freeze for half an hour.

6. Slice the square into 25 equally-sized bites.

7. Keep chilled until ready to enjoy.

Nutrition per Serving

Cals 60 | Fat 3g | Carbs 7.5g | Protein 1.5g

(18) Tuna Salad with Black Beans and Avocado

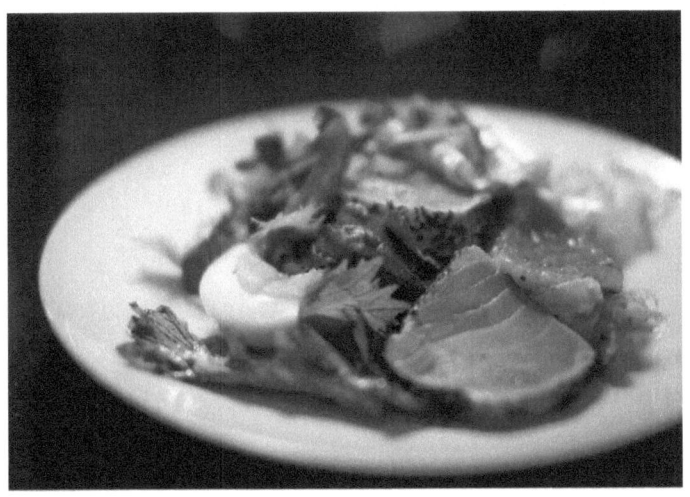

Enjoy this delicious tuna salad with crackers, on top of toast or even as a filling salad topper. Did you know that tuna is a great source of lean protein?

Yield: 2

Cooking Time: 5mins

List of Ingredients:

- 1 (5 ounce) can yellowfin tuna in oil (drained)
- ½ ripe avocado (peeled, pitted, mashed)
- ½ cup canned black beans (rinsed)
- 10 cherry tomatoes (halved)
- ¼ cup fresh cilantro (roughly chopped)
- Juice of ½ a medium lime
- Sea salt and black pepper

MMMMMMMMMMMMMMMMMMMMMMMMMMMMMMMMMM

Methods:

1. Add the tuna, avocado, and black beans to a bowl and stir to combine.

2. Add the tomatoes, cilantro, lime juice, and seasoning and stir again.

3. Serve with crackers, toast, or lettuce leaves.

Nutrition per Serving

Cals 250 | Fat 13g | Carbs 20g | Protein 17g

(19) Bouncing Banana Balls

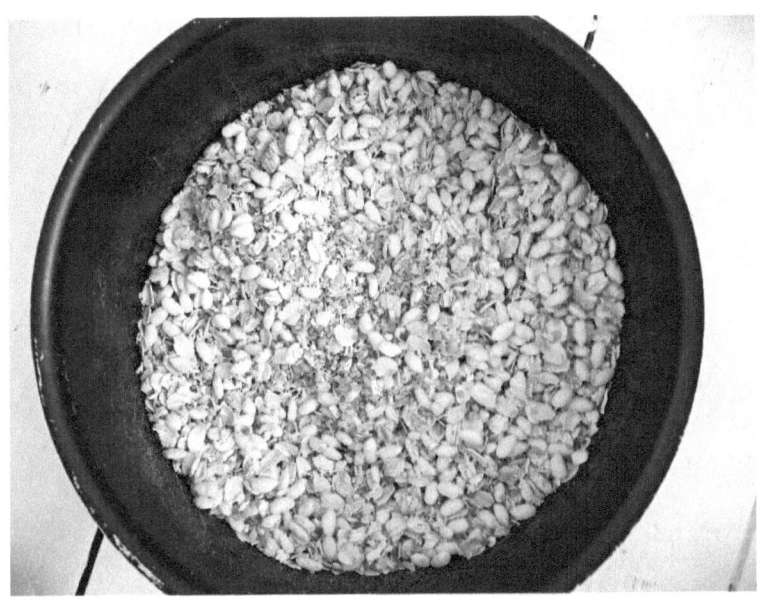

These tasty little balls will have you bouncing with energy! Keep them on hand for a much-needed boost.

Yield: 12

Cooking Time: 10mins

List of Ingredients:

- 1 scoop vanilla-flavored protein powder
- 1 cup oats
- 1 large, ripe banana (peeled, chopped)

MMMMMMMMMMMMMMMMMMMMMMMMMMMMMMMMMMMMMM

Methods:

1. Add the protein powder, and oats to a blender and blitz until finely chopped.

2. Add the banana and pulse until the dough comes together.

3. Roll the mixture into 12 equal balls and chill for an hour until firm.

4. Store in a sealed container in the refrigerator.

Nutrition per Serving

Cals 50 | Fat 0.5g | Carbs 8g | Protein 3g

(20) Spicy Avocado and Quinoa Muffins

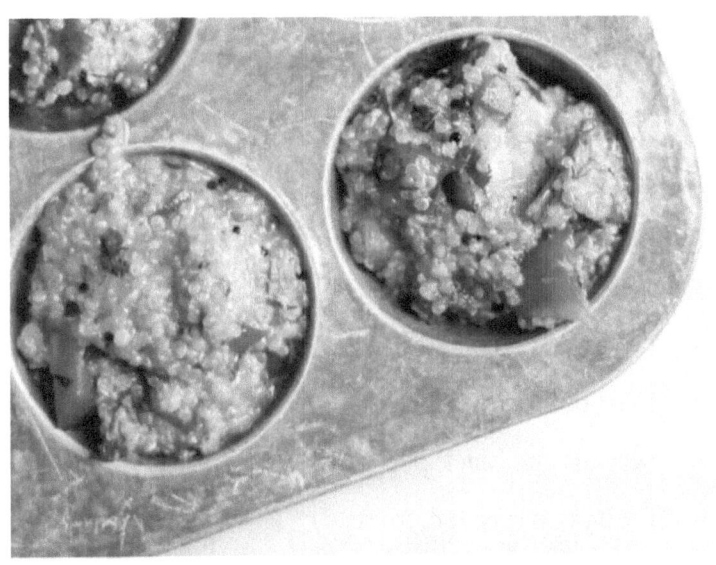

Did you know that quinoa is one of the most protein-rich foods in the world? It contains all 9 essential amino acids, as well as fiber, iron, and magnesium. Incorporate this delicious grain into your diet with these delicious spicy muffins.

Yield: 4

Cooking Time: 40mins

List of Ingredients:

- 2 cups water
- 1 cup quinoa (uncooked)
- Nonstick spray
- White of 3 eggs
- 3 eggs
- 2 tablespoons fresh cilantro (chopped)
- 1 cup baby spinach (chopped)
- ¼ cup red onion (peeled, diced)
- 1 avocado (peeled, pitted, diced)
- 1 red bell pepper (seeded, diced)
- Sea salt and black pepper
- 1 jalapeno (seeded, minced)

MMMMMMMMMMMMMMMMMMMMMMMMMMMMMMMMMM

Methods:

1. Bring the water to a boil in a saucepan and add the quinoa. Cook, while covered, for 15 minutes over low heat until the water completely absorbs. Take off the heat, fluff and allow to cool.

2. Preheat the main oven to 350 degrees F and spritz a 12-hole muffin tin with nonstick spray.

3. Beat the egg whites and eggs together in a large bowl. Add the cilantro, spinach, onion, avocado, bell pepper, seasoning, and jalapeno. Stir gently until well combined.

4. Fold in the quinoa.

5. Divide the mixture between the holes of the muffin tin and place in the oven. Cook for just over 20 minutes until set.

6. Allow to cool completely before serving.

7. Store in a sealed container in the refrigerator for up to a week.

Nutrition per Serving

Cals 115 | Fat 5g | Carbs 12.5g | Protein 5g

(21) Burrito in a Jar

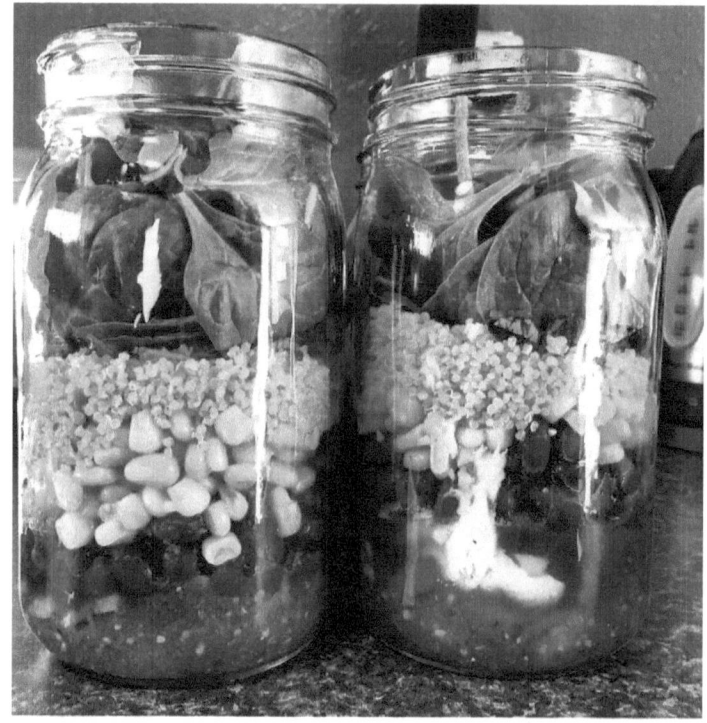

A tasty make-ahead snack in a jar, perfect for having on hand for a pre or post-workout protein-energy boost.

Yield: 4

Cooking Time: 1hour

List of Ingredients:

- 15 ounces canned black beans (rinsed)
- 1 cup tomato salsa
- 1 cup low-fat Cheddar cheese (grated)
- ½ cup fat-free sour cream

MMMMMMMMMMMMMMMMMMMMMMMMMMMMMMMMMMMMM

Methods:

1. Take 4 (½ pint) resealable jars.

2. Into each jar, layer a quarter of the black beans, followed by a quarter of the salsa, a quarter of the Cheddar, and 2 tablespoons of sour cream.

3. Seal the jars and keep chilled for up to 3 days.

Nutrition per Serving

Cals 190 | Fat 2g | Carbs 27g | Protein 15g

(22) Pistachio and Vanilla Cream Sandwich Cookies

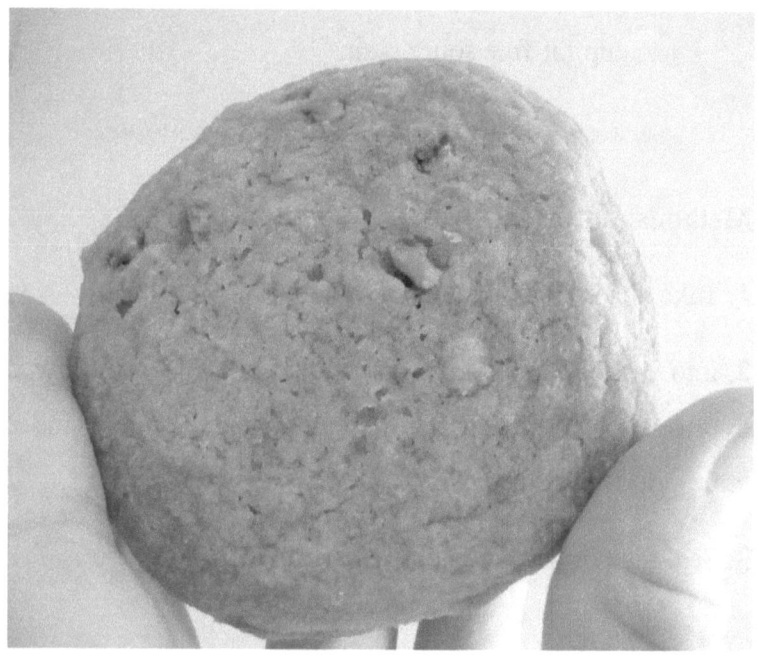

No-bake pistachio cookies are filled with a smooth vanilla 'cream' for a delicious sweet treat that you would never guess is gluten-free, dairy-free, vegan, high in protein, antioxidants, and iron!

Yield: 16

Cooking Time: 20mins

List of Ingredients:

Cookies:

- ½ cup shredded coconut
- 1 cup raw pistachios
- ¼ cup rolled oats (gluten-free)
- 1 tablespoon moringa powder
- 2 tablespoons pure maple syrup
- 1 teaspoon vanilla essence
- 1½ tablespoons water

Filling:

- ½ cup raw cashews
- 1 cup shredded coconut
- ¼ cup rolled oats (gluten-free)
- 1 teaspoon vanilla essence
- 2 tablespoons organic almond butter
- 1 tablespoon virgin coconut oil (melted)

MMMMMMMMMMMMMMMMMMMMMMMMMMMMMMMM

Methods:

1. Add the shredded coconut, pistachios, oats, moringa powder, maple syrup, vanilla essence, and water to a food processor and blitz until the mixture comes together.

2. Cover your work surface with plastic wrap and turn the dough out onto it, cover with another piece of plastic wrap.

3. Roll the dough into a ½" thick sheet. Cut 32 equally-sized discs from the dough, re-rolling as necessary.

4. Arrange the discs on a cookie sheet and freeze for several minutes.

5. In the meantime, make the filling, Add the cashews, coconut, oats, vanilla essence, almond butter, and melted coconut oil to a food processor and blitz until smooth.

6. Spread 16 of the frozen cookies with the vanilla filling and sandwich together with the remaining cookies.

7. Serve straight away or keep chilled until ready to enjoy.

Nutrition per Serving

Cals 135 | Fat 10g | Carbs 8.5g | Protein 3.5g

(23) Carrot Cake Chia Pudding

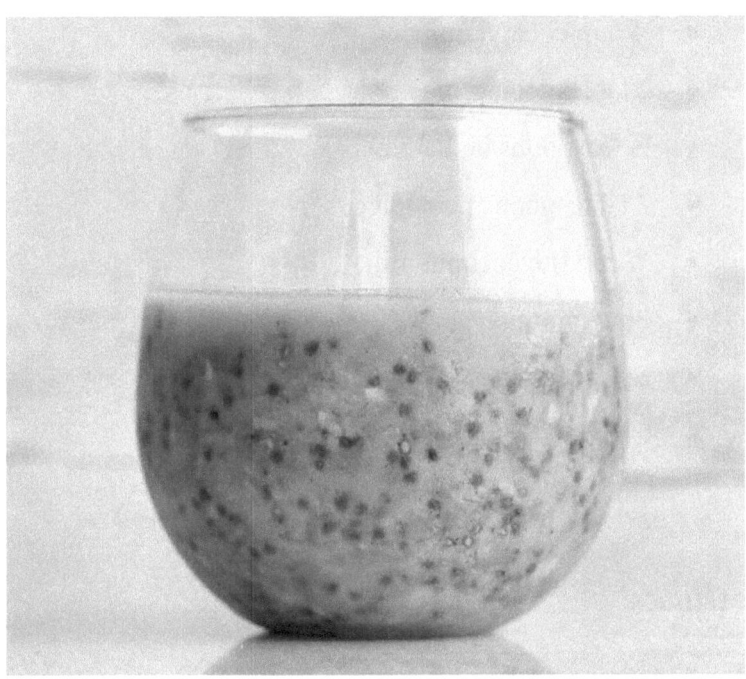

Don't be fooled by their tiny size; one of the most nutritious foods on the planet chia seeds are packed full of protein, fiber, micronutrients, and Omega-3 fatty acids!

Yield: 1

Cooking Time: 8hours 5mins

List of Ingredients:

- ¼ cup shredded carrot
- ¼ cup cooked quinoa
- 2 tablespoons chia seeds
- ½ teaspoons cinnamon
- 2 tablespoons hemp hearts
- ⅔ cup lite coconut milk
- Pinch nutmeg
- Chopped dates (for topping)
- Chopped walnuts (for topping)

MMMMMMMMMMMMMMMMMMMMMMMMMMMMMMMMMMM

Methods:

1. Add the carrot, quinoa, chia seeds, cinnamon, hemp hearts, coconut milk, and nutmeg in a resealable mason jar. Stir well, seal and chill overnight.

2. The following day, stir once more and top with chopped dates and walnuts.

Nutrition per Serving

Cals 625 | Fat 51g | Carbs 31g | Protein 20g

(24) Peanut Chicken Rainbow Salad Wraps

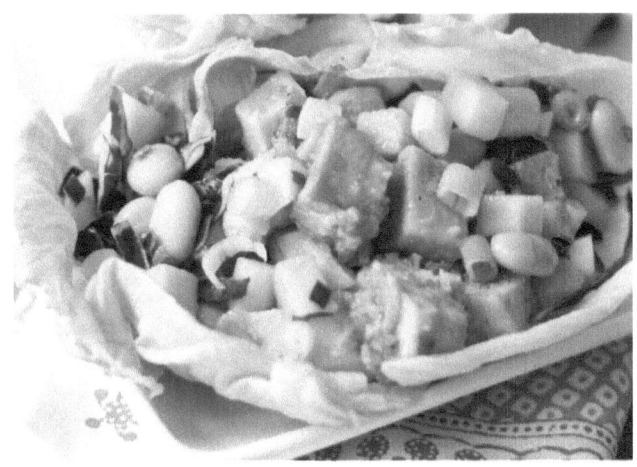

Crunchy fresh vegetables and chicken in a mouth-watering sauce all wrapped in a spinach tortilla make a delicious and filling snack that will help you to hit your daily protein goals.

Yield: 4

Cooking Time: 15mins

List of Ingredients:

Peanut Sauce:

- 2 tablespoons soy sauce
- ¼ cup organic smooth peanut butter
- 1 teaspoon fresh ginger (peeled, grated)
- 1 tablespoon rice wine vinegar
- 1 teaspoon organic honey
- 2 tablespoons warm water
- Dash hot sauce

Wraps:

- ¾ cup grated carrots
- ¾ cup red cabbage (shredded)
- 1 red bell pepper (seeded, julienned)
- 2 cups baby spinach
- ¼ cup scallions (diced)
- ¼ cup fresh cilantro (finely chopped)
- 1 pound cooked, chopped chicken breast
- 2 tablespoons peanuts (chopped)
- 2 (12") spinach tortillas

MMMMMMMMMMMMMMMMMMMMMMMMMMMMMMMMMMMM

Methods:

1. First, make the dressing. Add the soy sauce, peanut butter, ginger, vinegar, honey, water, and hot sauce in a small bowl and stir to combine. Set aside.

2. Divide the vegetables, chicken, and peanuts equally between the spinach tortillas and drizzle with the prepared dressing.

3. Fold the bottom of each tortilla up to cover the filling then fold in the left and right sides to make two wraps.

4. Slice in half and serve.

Nutrition per Serving

Cals 300 | Fat 12g | Carbs 31g | Protein 20g

(25) Cheesy Sausage and Egg Cups

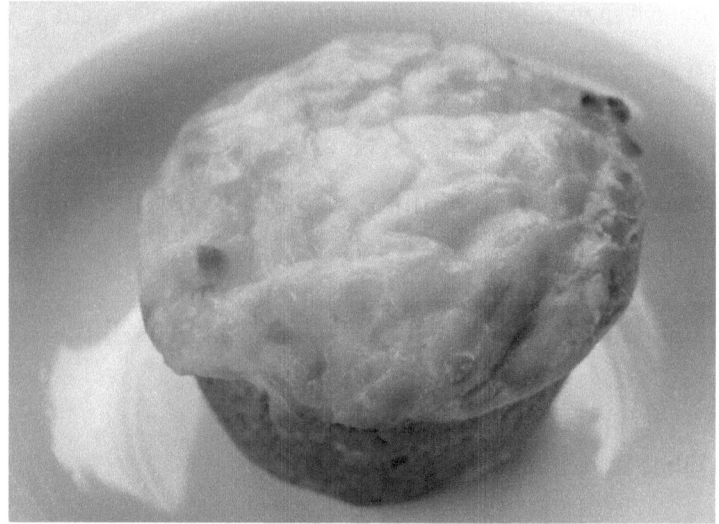

These cheesy sausage and egg cups are super tasty and satisfying. The ultimate low-carb snack to give you that much-needed boost before a big workout.

Yield: 12

Cooking Time: 25mins

List of Ingredients:

- Nonstick spray
- ½ cup almond milk (unsweetened)
- 8 eggs
- Black pepper
- ½ teaspoons kosher salt
- ⅓ cup coconut flour
- 1 cup Cheddar cheese (grated)
- ½ pound cooked chicken sausage (cooked)

MMMMMMMMMMMMMMMMMMMMMMMMMMMMMMMMMMMM

Methods:

1. Preheat the main oven to 400 degrees F and spritz a 12-hole muffin tin with nonstick spray.

2. Beat together the milk, eggs, black pepper, and kosher salt until combined.

3. Stir in the flour until incorporated, then fold in half of the Cheddar and all of the sausage.

4. Pour the mixture into the holes of the muffin tin, sprinkle over the remaining Cheddar and place in the oven. Bake for 15 minutes until the muffins puff up, and the eggs are completely cooked.

5. Enjoy warm.

Nutrition per Serving

Cals 140 | Fat 9g | Carbs 4.5g | Protein 10g

(26) Fully-Loaded Blueberry Oatmeal Cookies

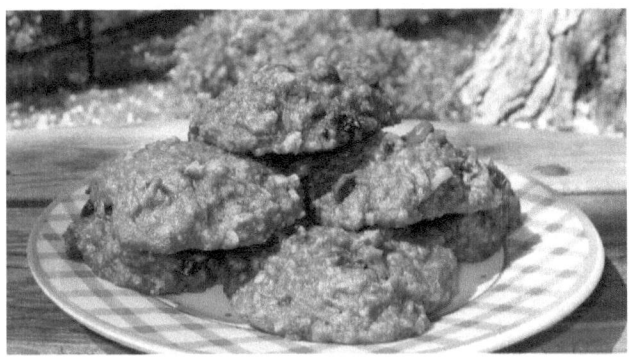

Just because you're trying to get into shape doesn't mean you have to miss out on your favorite treats! These fully-loaded, chewy cookies are bursting with blueberries, spices, nuts, and more importantly, Omega-3!

Yield: 8

Cooking Time: 30mins

List of Ingredients:

- ¼ cup coconut sugar
- 2 tablespoons coconut oil (melted)
- ½ teaspoons almond essence
- 1 overripe banana (peeled, mashed)
- ½ teaspoons vanilla essence
- ½ cup almond meal
- ¼ cup flaxseed meal
- ½ teaspoons cinnamon
- ½ teaspoons bicarb of soda
- ¼ teaspoons kosher salt
- 1 tablespoon chia seeds
- 1¼ cups oats
- ¼ cup walnuts (chopped)
- ½ cup fresh blueberries

MMMMMMMMMMMMMMMMMMMMMMMMMMMMMMMMMM

Methods:

1. Preheat the main oven to 350 degrees F. Cover a cookie sheet with parchment, set to one side.

2. Add the sugar, oil, almond essence, mashed banana, and vanilla essence to a bowl and beat until combined.

3. Add the almond meal, flaxseed meal, cinnamon, bicarb of soda, and salt stirring until incorporated.

4. Add the chia seeds and oats, stirring again.

5. Finally, fold in the walnuts and blueberries until evenly distributed.

6. Scoop a ¼ cup of cookie dough at a time and use hands to compact it into a tight ball. Place on the cookie sheet and gently press down to flatten.

7. Repeat with the remaining batter to form 8 large cookies.

8. Place in the oven and bake for approximately 15 minutes until golden.

9. Allow to cool completely before enjoying.

Nutrition per Serving

Cals 205 | Fat 12g | Carbs 22g | Protein 5g

(27) Cinnamon-Spiced Pancakes

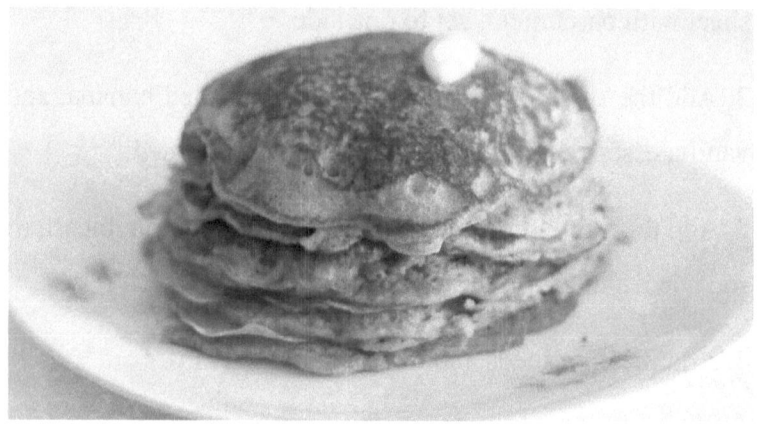

With just four ingredients, these fluffy little pancakes are both quick and delicious. What's more, they are high in protein and very low in fat. It doesn't get better than that!

Yield: 4

Cooking Time: 20mins

List of Ingredients:

- 1 cup egg whites
- 1 teaspoon calorie-free sweetener
- 2 tablespoons flaxseed (ground)
- Pinch cinnamon
- Nonstick spray
- 1 tablespoon organic creamy peanut butter (for topping)

MMMMMMMMMMMMMMMMMMMMMMMMMMMMMMMMMMMM

Methods:

1. Add the egg whites, sweetener, flaxseeds, and cinnamon to a blender. Blitz until combined.

2. Heat a skillet over moderate heat and spritz with nonstick spray.

3. Cook the batter as desired (either to make large or mini pancakes) flipping when the batter bubbles and the edges firm and then cooking for 2 minutes more until golden.

4. Serve the cooked pancakes with peanut butter.

Nutrition per Serving

Cals 120 | Fat 4g | Carbs 12g | Protein 10g

Chapter III - Protein Shakes

MMMMMMMMMMMMMMMMMMMMMMMMMMMMMMMMMMMM

(28) Orange Creamsicle Shake

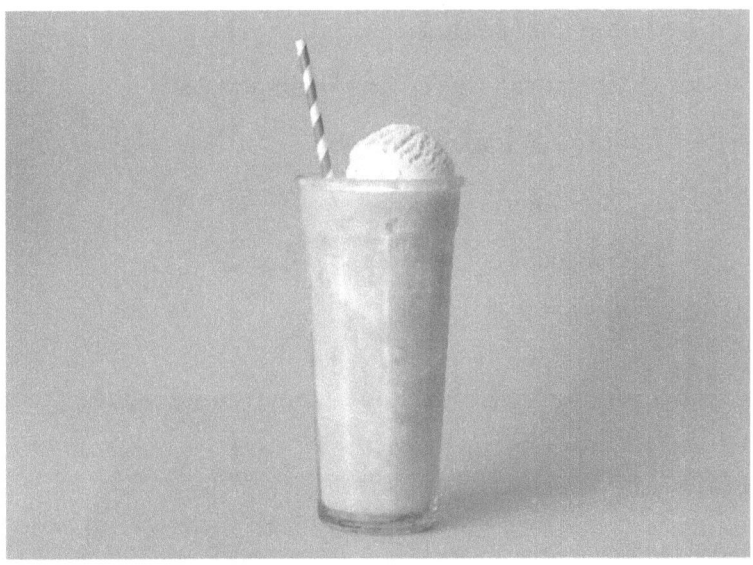

With a whopping 43g of protein per serving, this orange creamsicle shake is the most delicious and effective way to help you meet your daily protein goals!

Yield: 1

Cooking Time: 5mins

List of Ingredients:

- 3 ounces frozen orange juice concentrate
- ½ cup almond milk
- 2 scoops vanilla-flavor protein powder
- 1 teaspoon organic honey
- ½ cup water
- ½ banana (peeled, chopped, frozen)
- Few cubes of ice

MMMMMMMMMMMMMMMMMMMMMMMMMMMMMMMMMMMMM

Methods:

1. Add the juice concentrate, milk, protein powder, honey, water, and banana to a blender. Blitz until smooth.

2. Add the ice and pulse until no large shards remain.

3. Pour into a glass and enjoy.

Nutrition per Serving

Cals 490 | Fat 6g | Carbs 69g | Protein 43g

(29) Green Machine

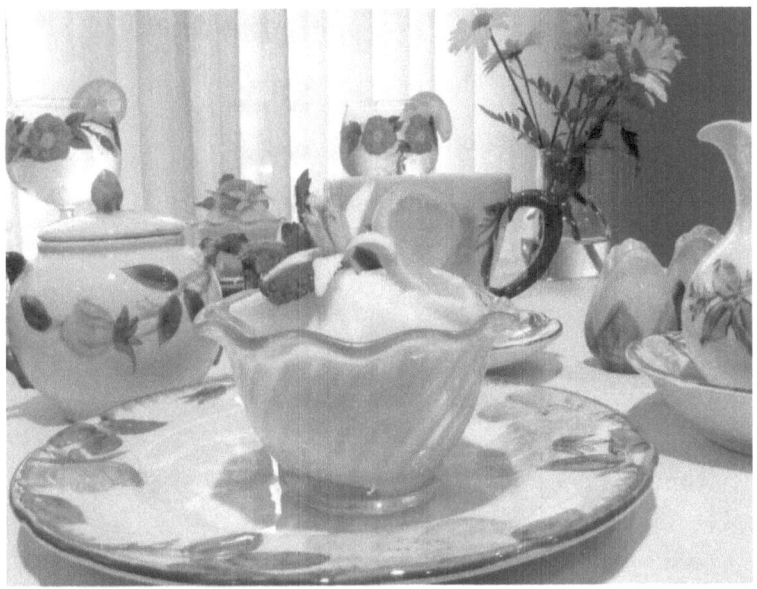

This tropical green smoothie will have you feeling like a machine, ready to smash that workout!

Yield: 1

Cooking Time: 5mins

List of Ingredients:

- ½ medium banana
- 2 scoops vanilla-flavor protein powder
- ½ cup frozen chopped pineapple
- 1 cup almond milk
- 1 cup frozen chopped peach
- 1 tablespoon flaxseed
- 2 cups kale

MMMMMMMMMMMMMMMMMMMMMMMMMMMMMMMMMMM

Methods:

1. Add the banana, protein powder, pineapple, milk, peach, flaxseed, and kale in a blender. Blitz until smooth.

2. Pour into glasses and serve.

Nutrition per Serving

Cals 550 | Fat 10.5g | Carbs 70g | Protein 48.5g

(30) Apple and Spirulina Crush

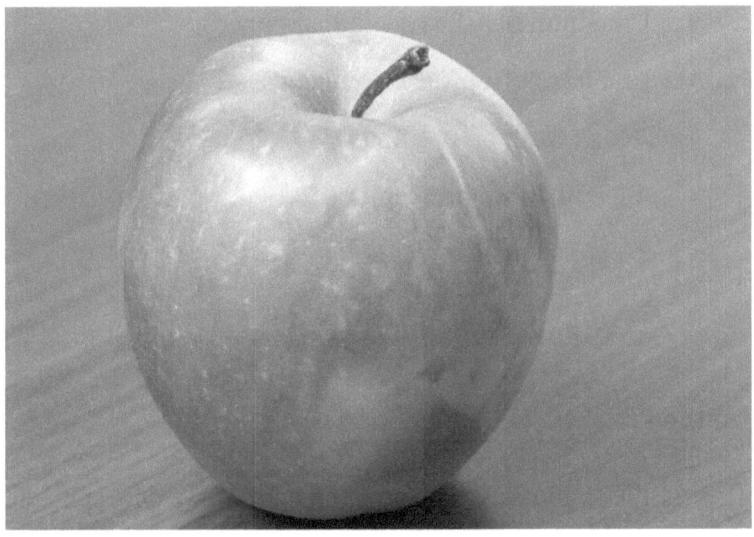

Spirulina is a natural plant-based protein, ideal for those looking for a more organic alternative to traditional protein powders. Drink this apple and spirulina iced crush as a post-workout refresher and detoxifier.

Yield: 2

Cooking Time: 5mins

List of Ingredients:

- 13 ounces organic apple juice
- 1 medium banana (peeled, chopped)
- 1 tablespoon spirulina powder
- 2 cups fresh baby spinach
- Juice of 2 medium lemons
- 2½ cups crushed ice

MMMMMMMMMMMMMMMMMMMMMMMMMMMMMMMMMMMMM

Methods:

1. Add the apple juice, banana, spirulina powder, spinach, lemon juice, and crushed ice in a blender. Blitz until smooth.

2. Pour into two glasses and serve.

Nutrition per Serving

Cals 95 | Fat 1g | Carbs 22g | Protein 4.5g

(31) Pumpkin Pie Protein Smoothie

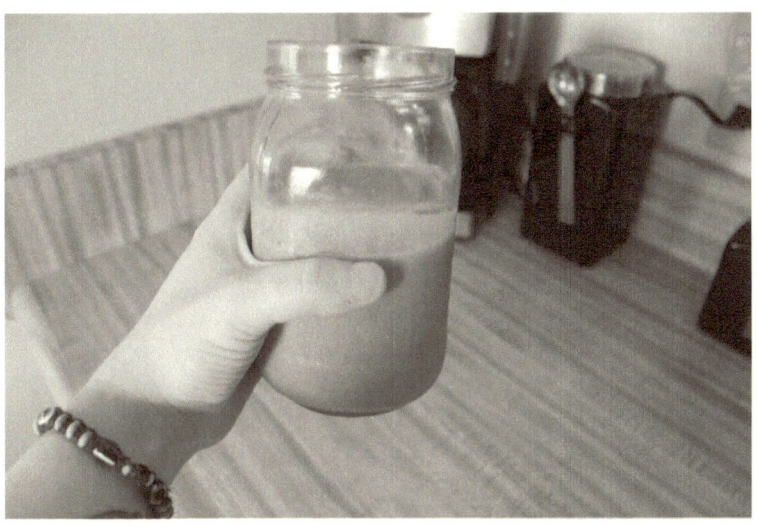

A holiday-inspired smoothie that will help to curb any dessert cravings while also giving your body that much-need punch of protein.

Yield: 1

Cooking Time: 5mins

List of Ingredients:

- 2 scoops vanilla-flavor protein powder
- ¼ teaspoons pumpkin pie spice
- 1 cup almond milk
- 3 tablespoons pureed pumpkin
- 1 banana (peeled, chopped, frozen)

MMMMMMMMMMMMMMMMMMMMMMMMMMMMMMMMMMMMMM

Methods:

1. Add the protein powder, pie spice, milk, pumpkin, and banana to a blender. Blitz until smooth.

2. Pour into a glass and enjoy.

Nutrition per Serving

Cals 295 | Fat 6g | Carbs 37g | Protein 27g

(32) Big Blue Booster

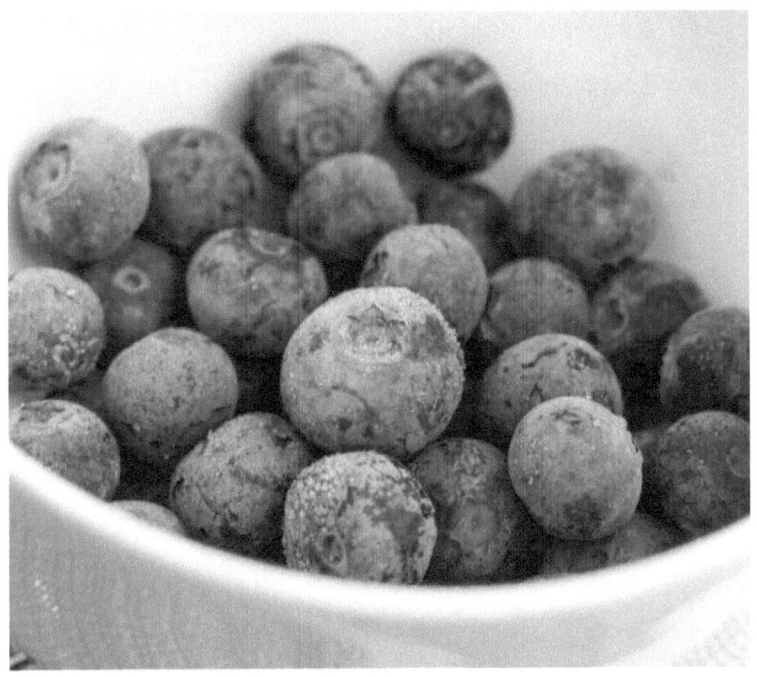

Blueberries are bursting with Vitamin K and C as well as manganese, fiber, and antioxidants not to mention refreshing, fruity flavor!

Yield: 1

Cooking Time: 5mins

List of Ingredients:

- ½ cup frozen blueberries
- 1 cup almond milk
- 1 tablespoon chia seeds
- 2 scoops vanilla-flavor protein powder
- ½ cup frozen chopped mango

MMMMMMMMMMMMMMMMMMMMMMMMMMMMMMMMMMM

Methods:

1. Add the blueberries, almond milk, chia seeds, protein powder, and mango to a blender. Blitz until smooth.

2. Pour into a glass and enjoy.

Nutrition per Serving

Cals 455 | Fat 11.5g | Carbs 47g | Protein 48.5g

(33) PB&J Protein Shake

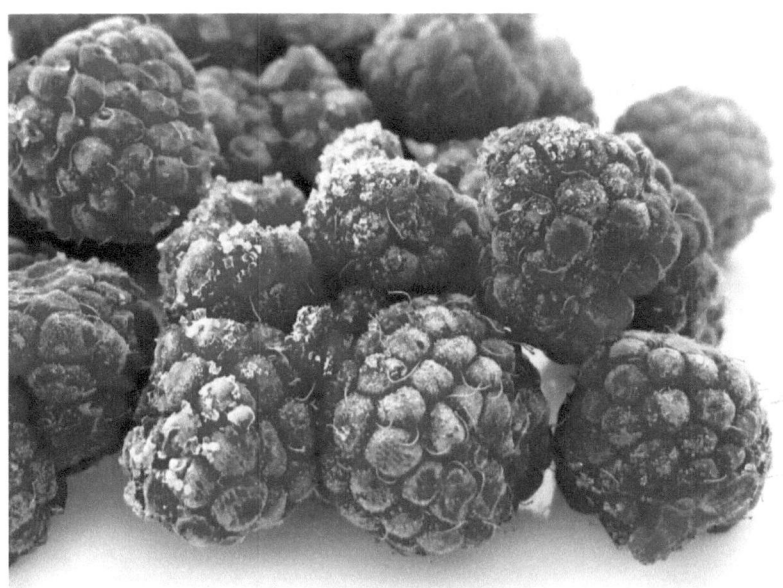

Get yourself fuelled up for your next workout with this super tasty PB&J protein shake.

Yield: 1

Cooking Time: 5mins

List of Ingredients:

- 2 scoops vanilla-flavor protein powder
- 1 cup almond milk
- 1 tablespoon organic smooth peanut butter
- ½ cup frozen raspberries

MMMMMMMMMMMMMMMMMMMMMMMMMMMMMMMMMMMM

Methods:

1. Add the protein powder, almond milk, peanut butter, and berries in a blender. Blitz until smooth.

2. Pour into a glass and enjoy.

Nutrition per Serving

Cals 315 | Fat 14g | Carbs 21g | Protein 30g

(34) Black Forest Cake Shake

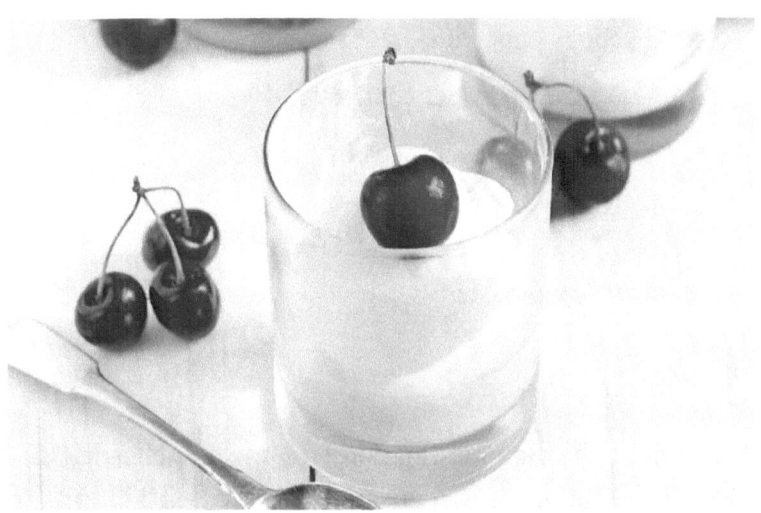

A delicious-tasting dessert inspired shake that also delivers a whopping dose of protein? Almost too good to be true!

Yield: 1

Cooking Time: 5mins

List of Ingredients:

- 1 cup almond milk
- 2 scoops chocolate-flavor protein powder
- 1 cup frozen sweet cherries
- 1 medium banana (peeled, chopped)
- Few cubes of ice

MMMMMMMMMMMMMMMMMMMMMMMMMMMMMMMMMMMMMM

Methods:

1. Combine the almond milk, protein powder, cherries, and banana and add to a blender; blitz until smooth.

2. Add the ice cubes and pulse until no large ice shards remain.

3. Pour into a glass and enjoy.

Nutrition per Serving

Cals 375 | Fat 4g | Carbs 53g | Protein 37g

(35) Mocha Shake

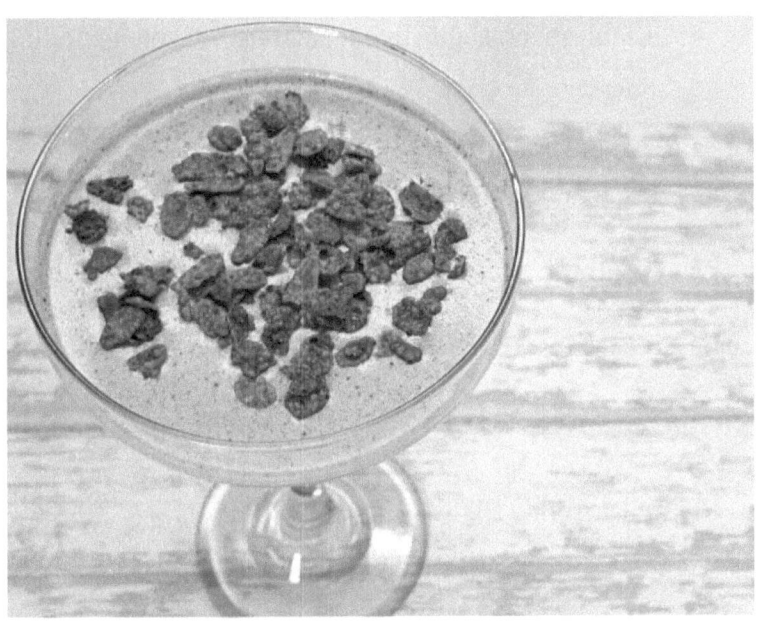

Get your caffeine fix, protein boost and satisfy chocolate cravings all at the same time with this delicious mocha shake.

Yield: 1

Cooking Time: 5mins

List of Ingredients:

- ½ cup almond milk
- 1 tablespoon sugar-free instant butterscotch pudding powder
- ½ cup strong-brewed coffee (chilled)
- 2 scoops chocolate-flavor protein powder
- 1 cup ice

MMMMMMMMMMMMMMMMMMMMMMMMMMMMMMMMMMMM

Methods:

1. Add the milk, pudding powder, coffee, and protein powder in a blender. Blitz until smooth.

2. Add the ice and pulse until no large shards remain.

3. Pour into a glass and enjoy.

Nutrition per Serving

Cals 160 | Fat 1.5g | Carbs 11g | Protein 25g

(36) Chilli-Spiked Mango Shake

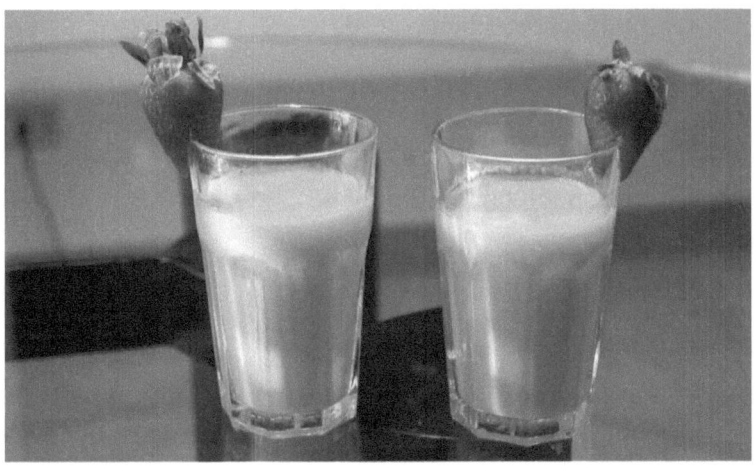

Chili is renowned for its metabolism boosting properties, whizz up this shake if you're trying to shift stubborn fat.

Yield: 2

Cooking Time: 5mins

List of Ingredients:

- 2 tablespoons goji berry powder
- 3 tablespoons hemp seeds
- 2½ cups chopped frozen mango
- 1½ cups organic, sugar-free apple juice
- 1 teaspoon hot chilli powder
- Juice of 1 medium lime
- 1 cup water

MMMMMMMMMMMMMMMMMMMMMMMMMMMMMMMMM

Methods:

1. Add the goji berry powder, hemp seeds, mango, apple juice, chili powder, lime juice, and water to a blender. Blitz until smooth.

2. Pour into two glasses and serve.

Nutrition per Serving

Cals 320 | Fat 8g | Carbs 61g | Protein 6g

(37) Matcha Green Tea Smoothie

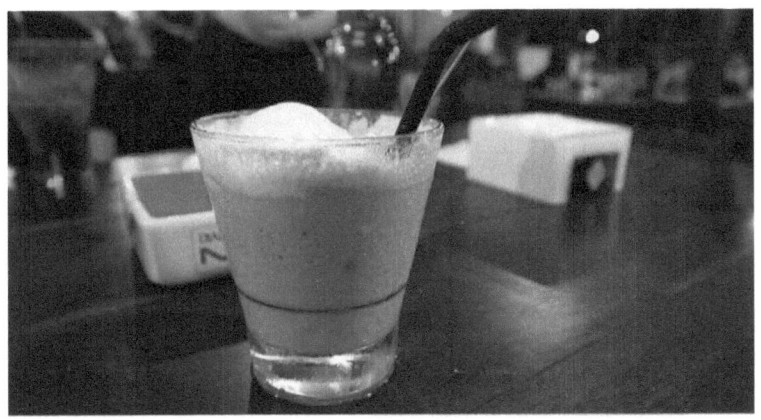

With high levels of protein, minerals, vitamins, antioxidants, and fiber, it is no wonder that matcha green tea was one of last year's biggest food trends. Get a taste of the action with this nutritious and delicious smoothie.

Yield: 4

Cooking Time: 5mins

List of Ingredients:

- 2 tablespoons matcha green tea powder
- 4½ cups almond milk
- 2 tablespoons almond flour
- 2 tablespoons hemp protein powder
- 4 Medjool dates (pitted)
- 2 tablespoons dried mulberries
- 1 tablespoon flaxseed meal
- 1 teaspoon zero-calorie sweetener
- 2 cups ice

MMMMMMMMMMMMMMMMMMMMMMMMMMMMMMMMMM

Methods:

1. Add the tea powder, milk, flour, protein powder, dates, mulberries, flaxseed meal, sweetener, and ice in a blender. Blitz until smooth.

2. Pour into four glasses and serve.

Nutrition per Serving

Cals 175 | Fat 8g | Carbs 18g | Protein 10g

(38) Coconut Macaroon Shake

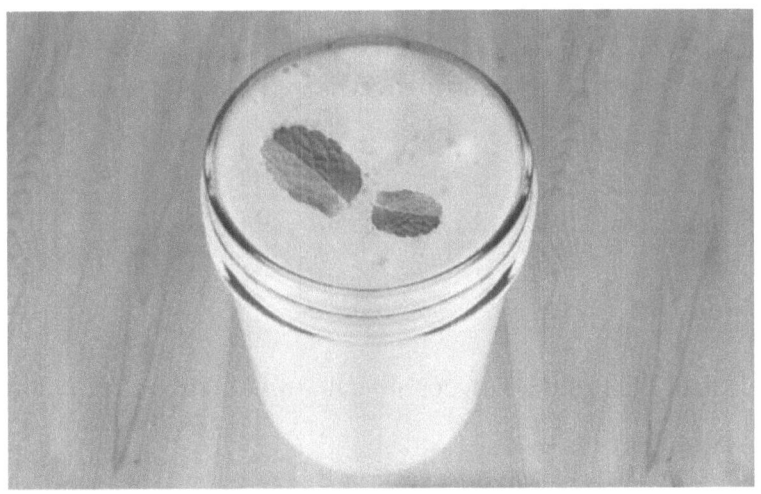

Four ingredients are all it takes to make this protein-packed shake that tastes just like your favorite coconut cookie.

Yield: 1

Cooking Time: 5mins

List of Ingredients:

- 2 scoops vanilla-flavor protein powder
- 1 cup coconut milk (not canned)
- ¼ cup toasted coconut flakes
- 1 cup ice

MMMMMMMMMMMMMMMMMMMMMMMMMMMMMMMMMMMM

Methods:

1. Add the protein powder, coconut milk, coconut flakes to a blender. Blitz until smooth.

2. Add the ice and pulse until no large shards remain.

3. Pour into a glass and enjoy.

Nutrition per Serving

Cals 300 | Fat 18g | Carbs 14g | Protein 25g

(39) Lean Green Shake

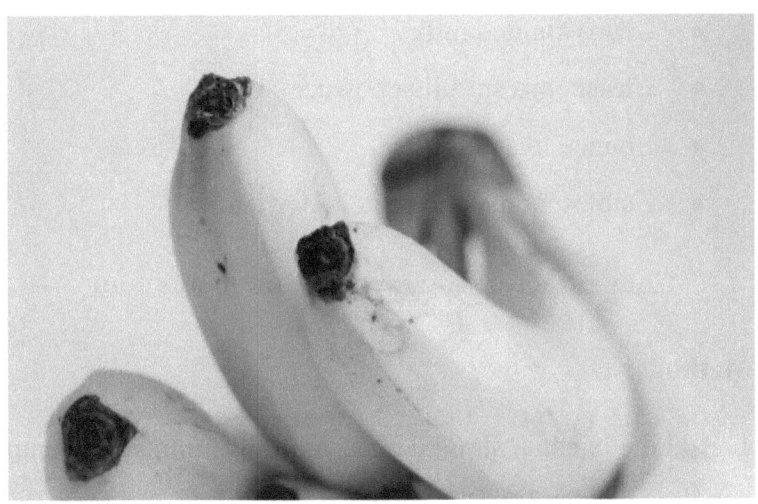

An all-natural shake that gets its protein from plant-based hemp powder, which contains an impressive 15g per serving!

Yield: 2

Cooking Time: 5mins

List of Ingredients:

- 1 banana (peeled, chopped, frozen)
- 2 cups almond milk
- 2 teaspoons spirulina powder
- 1 ounce fresh mint
- 1 tablespoon hemp protein powder

MMMMMMMMMMMMMMMMMMMMMMMMMMMMMMMMMMMM

Methods:

1. Add the banana, almond milk, spirulina, mint, and hemp powder in a blender. Blitz until smooth.

2. Pour into two glasses and enjoy.

Nutrition per Serving

Cals 265 | Fat 10g | Carbs 25g | Protein 20g

(40) Key Lime Pie Shake

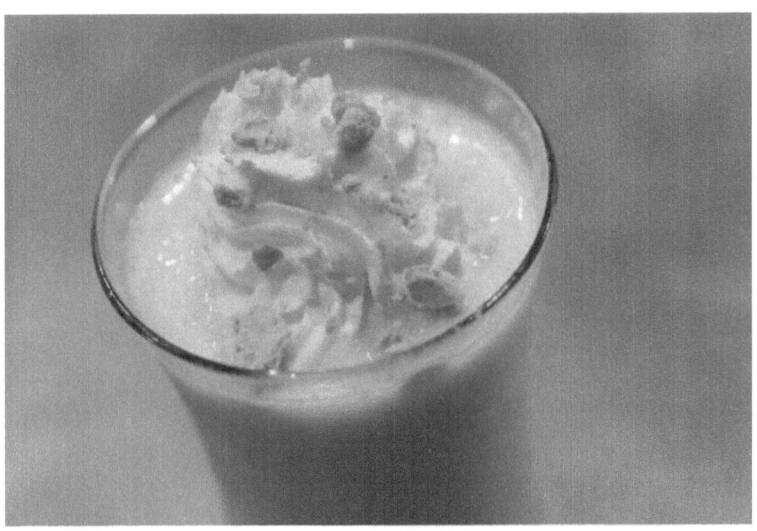

A sweet and zesty high-calorie protein shake that tastes like dessert in a glass. An ideal meal replacement shake for those busy days, or times when you're trying to cut a few pounds. What's not to love!?

Yield: 1

Cooking Time: 5mins

List of Ingredients:

- ½ cup almond milk
- 2 scoops vanilla-flavor protein powder
- 1 tablespoon key lime juice
- 1 banana (peeled, chopped, frozen)
- ½ teaspoons pure maple syrup
- Zest of 1 key lime
- 1 cup ice

MMMMMMMMMMMMMMMMMMMMMMMMMMMMMMMMMMMM

Methods:

1. Add the milk, protein powder, key lime juice, banana, maple syrup, and lime zest to a blender. Blitz until smooth.

2. Add the ice and pulse until no large shards remain.

3. Pour into a glass and enjoy.

Nutrition per Serving

Cals 700 | Fat 16g | Carbs 71g | Protein 83g

About the Author

A native of Indianapolis, Indiana, Valeria Ray found her passion for cooking while she was studying English Literature at Oakland City University. She decided to try a cooking course with her friends and the experience changed her forever. She enrolled at the Art Institute of Indiana which offered extensive courses in the culinary Arts. Once Ray dipped her toe in the cooking world, she never looked back.

When Valeria graduated, she worked in French restaurants in the Indianapolis area until she became the head chef at one of the 5-star establishments in the area. Valeria's attention to taste and visual detail caught the eye of a local business person who expressed an interest in publishing her recipes. Valeria began her secondary career authoring cookbooks and e-books which she tackled with as much talent and gusto as her first career. Her passion for food leaps off the page of her books which have colourful anecdotes and stunning pictures of dishes she has prepared herself.

Valeria Ray lives in Indianapolis with her husband of 15 years, Tom, her daughter, Isobel and their loveable Golden Retriever, Goldy. Valeria enjoys cooking special dishes in her large, comfortable kitchen where the family gets involved in preparing meals. This successful, dynamic chef is an inspiration to culinary students and novice cooks everywhere.

●●●●●●●●●●●●●●●●●●●●

Author's Afterthoughts

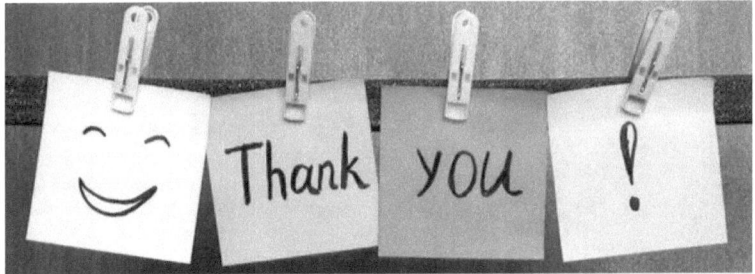

Thank you for Purchasing my book and taking the time to read it from front to back. I am always grateful when a reader chooses my work and I hope you enjoyed it!

With the vast selection available online, I am touched that you chose to be purchasing my work and take valuable time out of your life to read it. My hope is that you feel you made the right decision.

I very much would like to know what you thought of the book. Please take the time to write an honest and informative review on Amazon.com. Your experience and opinions will be of great benefit to me and those readers looking to make an informed choice.

With much thanks,

Valeria Ray